Update Gastroenterology 2000

Barrett's esophagus, colon cancer and tumor imaging

John Libbey Eurotext
127, avenue de la République
92120 Montrouge
Tél. : 33 (0) 1 46 73 06 60
e-mail : contact@john-libbey-eurotext.fr
http://www.john-libbey-eurotext.fr

John Libbey and Company Ltd
Collier House,
163-169 Brompton Road, Knightsbridge
London SW3 1 PY, England
Tel. : 44 (0) 20 75 81 24 49

CIC Edizioni Internazionali
Corso Trieste 42
00198 Roma, Italia
Tel. : 39 06 841 26 73

© John Libbey Eurotext, 2000
ISBN : 2-7420-0346-0

Il est interdit de reproduire intégralement ou partiellement le présent ouvrage - loi du 11 mars 1957 - sans autorisation de l'éditeur ou du Centre Français du Copyright, 6 *bis*, rue Gabriel-Laumain, 75010 Paris.

Update Gastroenterology 2000

Barrett's esophagus, colon cancer and tumor imaging

Edited by
R. Arnold, J.P. Galmiche

Postgraduate Course 2000
Brussels, November 25

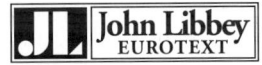

Contents

Foreword
R. Arnold, J.-P. Galmiche IX

I – Reflux esophagitis and Barrett's esophagus

LA-classification: pathophysiological and clinical relevance
L. Lundell 3

An update on the pathogenesis of Barrett's esophagus
P. Sharma 11

Surveillance of Barrett's esophagus: to screen or not to screen?
G.N.J. Tytgat 21

Barrett's esophagus: new endoscopic strategies in case of dysplasia and early cancer
C. Ell 29

II – Recent developments in gastro-intestinal oncology: colon cancer

Colon cancer screening
M.H. Vatn, G. Hoff, E. Thiis-Evensen 35

Primary prophylaxis of colon cancer: what is established?
M. Classen, E. Frimberger 47

The adjuvant treatment of colon cancer
E. Van Cutsem 57

Advanced colorectal cancer
J.M.G.H. van Riel 67

III – Cost-effective strategies in tumor staging and imaging

Staging and imaging of esophageal and gastric carcinoma
A. Sendler, H.J. Stein, J.R. Siewert 77

Staging and imaging of pancreatic cancer
K. Z'graggen, B.M. Schmied, H. Friess, M.W. Büchler 85

Staging and imaging of liver tumors
J. Gournay, B. Buecher, S. Monat 93

CT imaging of colonic tumors: hydro-CT and virtual colonoscopy
P.-J. Valette, J.-C. Saurin, P. Fouque, D. Marion 119

Laparoscopy: revival of an old technique?
A. Eickhoff, A.R.J. Schneider, J.C. Arnold, J.F. Riemann 129

List of contributors

Arnold J.-C., Medical Department C, Klinikum Ludwigshafen, Bremserstr. 79, D-67063 Ludwigshafen, Germany.

Büchler M.W., Department of Visceral and Transplantation Surgery, Inselspital, University of Bern, Murtenstr. 35, CH-3010 Bern, Switzerland.

Buecher B., Department of Gastroenterology and Hepatology, Centre Hospitalier Universitaire de Nantes, 44093 Nantes Cedex, France.

Classen M., Department of Internal Medicine II, Technical University, Ismaningen Street 2, D-81675 Munich, Germany.

Eickhoff A., Medical Department C, Klinikum Ludwigshafen, Bremserstr. 79, D-67063 Ludwigshafen, Germany.

Ell C., Department of Internal Medicine II, Gastroenterology, Dr. Horst Schmidt Klinik, Ludwig-Erhant Str. 100, D-65199 Wiesbaden, Germany.

Fouque P., Département des Spécialités Digestives, Hôpital Édouard-Herriot, place d'Arsonval, 69003 Lyon, France.

Friess H., Department of Visceral and Transplantation Surgery, Inselspital, University of Bern, Murtenstr. 35, CH-3010 Bern, Switzerland.

Frimberger E., Department of Internal Medicine II, Technical University, Ismaningen Street 2, D-81675 Munich, Germany.

Gournay J., Department of Gastroenterology and Hepatology, Centre Hospitalier Universitaire de Nantes, 44093 Nantes Cedex, France.

Hoff G., Medical Department, Telemark Central hospital, Skien, Norway.

Lundell L., Department of Surgery, Sahlgrenska University Hospital, S-41345 Gothenburg, Sweden.

Marion D., Service de Radiologie, Hôtel-Dieu, place de l'Hôpital, 69003 Lyon, France.

Monat S., Department of Gastroenterology and Hepatology, Centre Hospitalier Universitaire de Nantes, 44093 Nantes Cedex, France.

Riemann J.-F., Medical Department C, Klinikum Ludwigshafen, Bremserstr. 79, D-67063 Ludwigshafen, Germany.

Saurin J.-C., Service de Radiologie, Hôtel-Dieu, place de l'Hôpital, 69003 Lyon, France.

Schmied B.M., Department of Visceral and Transplantation Surgery, Inselspital, University of Bern, Murtenstr. 35, CH-3010 Bern, Switzerland.

Schneider A.R.J., Medical Department C, Klinikum Ludwigshafen, Bremserstr. 79, D-67063 Ludwigshafen, Germany.

Sendler A., Chirurgische Klinik und Poliklinik, Klinikum rechts der Isan der TU München, Ismaninger Str. 22, D-81675 München, Germany.

Sharma P., University of Kansas School of Medicine, Veterans Affairs Medical Center, 4801 E. Lindwood Blvd, Kansas City, mo 64128-2295, USA.

Siewert J.R., Chirurgische Klinik und Poliklinik, Klinikum rechts der Isan der TU München, Ismaninger Str. 22, D-81675 München, Germany.

Stein H.J., Chirurgische Klinik und Poliklinik, Klinikum rechts der Isan der TU München, Ismaninger Str. 22, D-81675 München, Germany.

Thiis-Evensen E., Medical Department, Telemark Central hospital, Skien, Norway.

Tytgat G.N.J., Academic Medical Center, Department of Gastroenterology and Hepatology, Meibergdreef 9, 1105 A2, Amsterdam Zuidoost, The Netherlands.

Valette P.-J., Département des Spécialités Digestives, Hôpital Édouard-Herriot, place d'Arsonval, 69003 Lyon, France.

Van Cutsem E., Department of Internal Medicine, University Hospital Gasthuisberg, Herestraat 49, B-3000 Leuven, Belgium.

Van Riel J.M.G.H., Department of Clinical Oncology, Free University Hospital, PO BOX 7057, 1007 MB Amsterdam, The Netherlands.

Vatn M.H., Medical Department, Riks-Hospitalet, University Hospital, N-0027 Oslo, Norway.

Z'graggen K., Department of Visceral and Transplantation Surgery, Inselspital, University of Bern, Murtenstr. 35, CH-3010 Bern, Switzerland.

Foreword

We welcome you to the EAGE Postgraduate Course 2000. The European Association of Gastroenterology and Endoscopy (EAGE) provides – as in the preceding years – on the eve of the United European Gastroenterology Week the opportunity for comprehensive education in important and topical issues in Gastroenterology. This year's course is designed to give an update in three important topics: reflux esophagitis and Barrett's esophagus, gastro-intestinal oncology and tumor imaging.

Barrett's esophagus is a pre-malignant condition for adenocarcinoma of the distal esophagus and of the gastroesophageal junction. Interestingly, only part of GERD patients develop Barrett's esophagus. Identification of simple markers that would allow stratification of patients that are at risk for the development of Barrett's esophagus would be of utmost importance and could eliminate the need for endoscopy in all patients with GERD. Therefore, the most relevant recent developments in our understanding of the pathophysiology, diagnosis, treatment and surveillance of Barrett's esophagus will be discussed during the first part of the Course.

Oncology is – as everybody agrees – one of the most important fields of interest in the world. Unfortunately, at least in some countries of Europe, gastroenterologists are only involved in screening and diagnosis but not in the management of patients with malignant disorders of the GI-tract. The organizers of this Course are convinced that for many reasons gastroenterologists should gain the expertise to manage patients with malignant conditions and that this expertise should not be restricted to local (endoscopic) treatment modalities. Therefore, the second part of the Course is devoted to aspects of screening, prophylaxis and medical treatment of colon cancer including chemotherapy.

In the third part, aspects of tumor staging and imaging will be discussed. This important issue of diagnosis of malignant conditions has relevant socio-economic consequences. Therefore, cost-effective strategies have to be defined which – on the one hand – recognize the latest developments in tumor imaging and define – on the other hand – the most cost-sparing approaches to select patients for the available treatment modalities.

A large group of international authorities has been invited and agreed to participate in the panel of speakers of the Course. The organizers acknowledge their tremendous efforts to contribute to the success of this Course by writing articles for the syllabus and to give important oral contributions to the different aspects of the Course.

Rudolf Arnold and Jean-Paul Galmiche
Course Directors

I

Reflux esophagitis and Barrett's esophagus

LA-classification: pathophysiological and clinical relevance

Lars Lundell

Department of Surgery, Sahlgrenska University Hospital, Gothenburg, Sweden

Gastroesophageal reflux disease is expressed in clinical practice in a variety of presentations. Endoscopy remains the choice investigation to make the diagnosis of reflux esophagitis and grading of its severity. Despite the fact that the lesions of the squamous epithelium may have a characteristic endoscopic appearance, these lesions can occur transiently or even be absent in severely symptomatic patients [1-3]. The endoscopic appearance of mucosal breaks has therefore a high specificity but lack sensitivity for GORD, since the endoscopic findings in reflux disease range from no or minimal changes to severe circumferential mucosal breaks with deep ulcerations and complications such as strictures and columnar lined esophagus [4]. Data indicate that the clinical response to treatment and the subsequent prognosis are dependent on the severity of these mucosal lesions. It is therefore important to classify and adequately assess the severity with which the mucosal breaks are affecting the esophagus [5]. Until recently this has been a significant problem in terms of lack of endoscopic classification systems which have been adequately assessed and validated. With respect to esophagitis, the situation was such that in fact we did not lack endoscopic classification for the severity but on the other hand had too many such systems. A survey of existing work indicated that there were more than 30 such systems documented in the literature [6]. This chaotic area was not likely to be helped by adapting an existing system or by developing another new system with the expectation that previous systems would be abounded. One of the most significant problems with the previously existing and used classification system was that virtually all existing systems are based on visual observations that have not yet been assessed for reproducibility.

Los Angeles grading of esophagitis

An international working group, which is supported by the World Organisation of Gastroenterology (OMGE), has been operational to define, evaluate and validate an endoscopic classification system for esophagitis. The working group developed and proposed the Los Angeles classification system in 1994 and reported its first evaluation of the criteria used [6]. The system was so named because it was presented at the Los Angeles World Congress of Gastroenterology. In the working group, agreement was reached on the definition of a mucosal break to be: an area of slough or an area of erythema with a discrete lined demarcation from the adjacent more normal looking mucosa. The group has continued to meet regularly in order to evaluate the proposed Los Angeles classification and as a result of these discussions has agreed that the definitive version [7] of this classification should be as given in *table I*. The members of the working group realised that it is sometimes difficult to determine confidently whether a mucosal break is completely circumferential or not. The change of grade D from fully circumferential to involvement of more than 75% of the circumference has required a matching modification of the definition of grade C.

Table I. The LA classification-system for the endoscopic assessment of reflux esophagitis (from [7]).

Grade A	Grade B
One (or more) mucosal break no longer than 5 mm, that does not extend between the tops of two mucosal folds.	One (or more) mucosal break more than 5 mm long, that does not extend between the tops of two mucosal folds.
Grade C	**Grade D**
One (or more) mucosal break that is continuous between the tops of two or more mucosal folds, but which involves less than 75% of the circumference.	One (or more) mucosal break which involves more than 75% of the esophageal circumference.

Methodology

A huge number of endoscopists from different countries and continents have participated. Both trained endoscopists, defined as those who had performed less than 500 upper GI endoscopies, and experts who had performed more than 3,000 upper GI endoscopies were invited to participate. We were unable to reveal any significant differences in outcome between these groups. Each participant received either a video tape which contained edited recordings of endoscopic images or still images. The full range of severity of reflux esophagitis was covered by the recordings. Endoscopists used a detailed worksheet, which was developed by the working group. The sheet scored from the full range of findings relevant to the evaluation of an esophagitis classification system according to predefined criteria [6, 8]. The most widely used coefficient of agreement in clinical studies, the Kappa statistics, was used in its original version in order to evaluate the degree of agreement among the observers. The range of possible values for Kappa is from -1 which indicates total disagreement, to +1 which is reached with perfect agreement. Agreement by chance alone gives a value of 0. Though far from perfect, values as low as 0.4 are considered to indicate acceptable agreement [9].

Esophageal pH-monitoring

The patients were recruited into the study if they had had heartburn as the main symptoms for at least 6 months or if their major symptom was acid regurgitation, abdominal pain or discomfort in association with heartburn. The patients scored their reflux induced symptoms in a structured manner during the last two days before involvement into the study and endoscopy was carried out and graded according to the suggested LA classification system. Before entry into the therapeutic trial, ambulatory, 24 h pH-monitoring was carried out with a monocristalline antimony electrode positioned 5 cm above the oral margin of the lower esophageal sphincter [10, 11].

Clinical studies

Patients with upper GI discomfort were recruited from primary care settings. The patients were screened for reflux symptoms by use of a questionnaire which had been developed for the diagnosis of symptomatic reflux disease and which focused especially on objective recognition of heartburn and on exacerbating or relieving factors. At endoscopy, patients with LA grade D esophagitis, columnar lined esophagus or peptic strictures were excluded from further involvement in the study. Complete endoscopic and clinical data were available whereupon patients were randomised to treatment. Patients without mucosal breaks were randomised to omeprazole either 20 or 10 mg daily or to placebo and those who had mucosal breaks had omeprazole either 10 or 20 mg daily. Treatment was given for 4 weeks under double blind conditions. All patients in whom symptoms were relieved at 4 or 8 weeks entered a follow-up period without treatment for up to 6 months exciting the study if their symptoms relapsed according to predefined criteria before that time [12, 13].

Intra-observer agreement

Severe complications

Severe complications of reflux disease (ulcer, stricture or columnar line mucosa) were noted by the majority of observers in approximately 1/4 of the observations made. These changes were reliably recorded, and among experienced endoscopists reviewing still images, Kappa values were high for ulcer (0.92), stricture (0.8) or columnar lined esophagus (0.82). Observations made by endoscopists under training were slightly less homogenous but still well within limits of acceptability. The investigators were also able to assess tongues of columnar metaplasia as well as those cases in which the metaplastic epithelium had a circumferential extent.

On the other hand, the investigator was specifically asked to assess the number and depth of ulcers, with an ulcer being defined as a mucosal break greater than 3 mm deep. Reliable judgement of the presence of an ulcer was not achieved as this assessment had a Kappa value of -0.01 and a corresponding Kappa value for the counting of the number of ulcers reached only -0.02.

Minimal changes

The presence and absence of minimal endoscopic changes as listed in *table II* was evaluated close to the esophago-gastric mucosal junction. There was no agreement on the presence or absence of these findings [14-17].

Table II. Reporting of esophageal minimal changes (from [7]).

Endoscopic features	Kappa values (CI)
• Reddening of the cardia	0.09 (0-0.29)
• Erythema of the SC junction	0 (-0.08-0.06)
• Friability of the SC junction	0.04 (0-0.25)
• Blurring of the SC junction	0.08 (0-0.22)
• Diffuse erythema of the esophagus	0.08 (0-0.28)
• Patchy erythema of the esophagus	0 (-0.07-0.09)
• Increased vascularity	0 (0-0.09)
• Edema, accentuated folds	0 (-0.02-0.15)

Mucosal breaks. Intra-observer agreement

As illustrated in the figures two categories were reliably identified and there was total (*figure 1* and *figure 2*) involvement of the entire circumference by the mucosal breaks with a Kappa value of 0.59 and the presence or absence of a mucosal break with a total involvement confined to at least 1 fold (Kappa value 0.84). Agreement on the presence or absence of mucosal break in a second intra-observer variability study indicated an intra observer agreement that was fair with a Kappa value of 0.4. The presence of multiple mucosal breaks (2 or more), that extended between 2 folds, was assessed with similar accuracy.

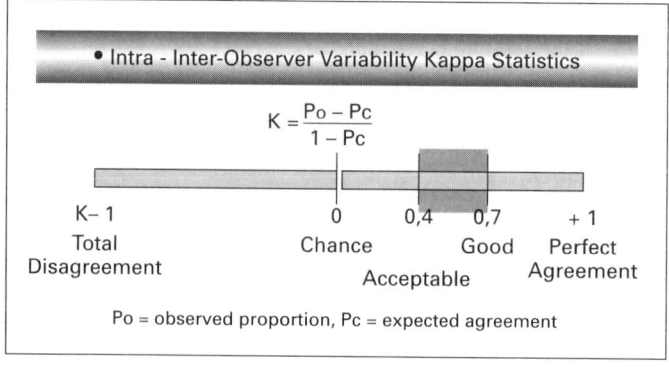

Figure 1. Validation of classification systems.

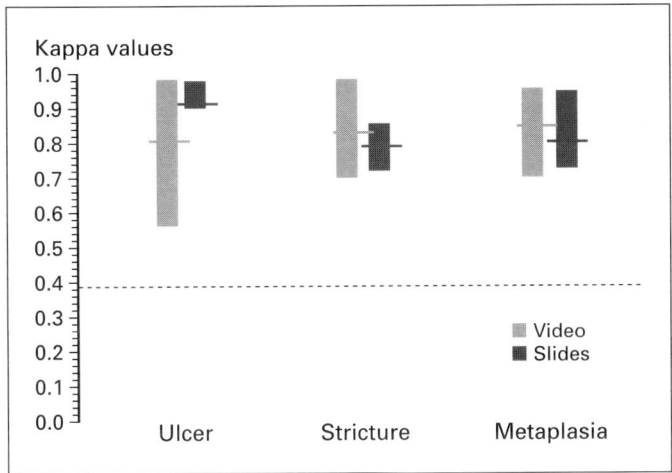

Figure 2. Observer agreement on the assessment of esophagitis (from [6]).

Functional and clinical correlates

Esophageal pH monitoring and symptom assessment were completed according to the protocol. There was a significant relation between the LA classification grade and the 24 h esophageal acid exposure values ($p < 0.01$) *(figure 3)*. There was also a significant correlation between pretreatment symptom severity and endoscopic grading of mucosal breaks. Consequently the severity of heartburn correlated significantly with the pretreatment endoscopic grading ($p < 0.01$). After 4 weeks treatment with omeprazole 10 mg daily, there was a gradation of endoscopic healing rates from 77% in grade A patients to only 20% in grade C patients. Symptomatic relapse after initial short-term treatment occurred in 83% of the patients during a 6 months follow-up period. The proportion of patients still in clinical remission during the 6 months showed a significant relationship to the pretreatment LA classification grade of the mucosal breaks. When the symptoms relapse, curves specifically compared the difference in the slopes between grade A patients *versus* normal reached a p-value of 0.04, normal *versus* grade A + B + C, a p-value of 0.002, and grade C *versus* the others a p-value of 0.003.

Concluding remarks

A useful endoscopic classification of reflux disease must fulfil a certain number of criteria. It should identify lesions specific for GORD with high accuracy and minimal inter- observer variability. The identification of lesions should not be dependent on technical developments within the field of fibreoptic technology and the classification should minimise the problem of misinterpretation of the extent of the lesion. It should also describe each lesion exactly, irrespective of the coexistence of other lesions. An important feature is

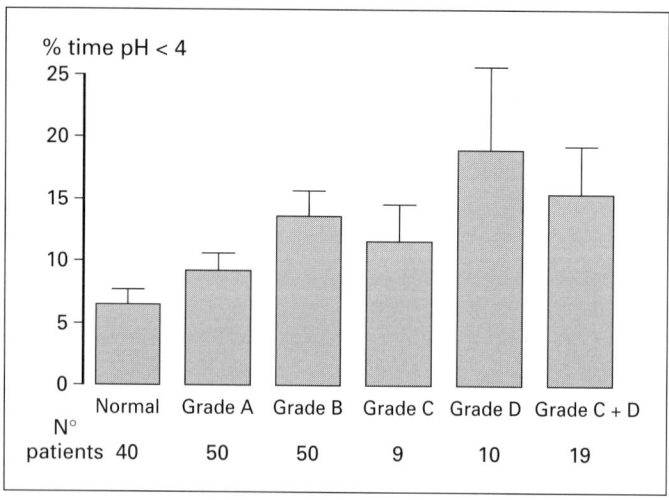

Figure 3. Acid reflux parameters as related to endoscopic grading of mucosal breaks (from [7]).

also to allow a practical collection of data and description of all concomitantly existing lesions and each grade of esophagitis should be distinct enough to avoid overlap. It is also important that the endoscopic classification can be easily memorised and provide a standardised, generally accepted and comprehensive, description of the disease specific features while differentiating clearly among minimal changes, mucosal breaks and complications. This system should also distinguish reversible from irreversible lesions.

The LA classification system was developed with the intention to provide a clinically relevant stratification of the severity of esophagitis. Despite the lack of validation of other esophagitis classification systems there is considerable amount of data indicating that these recognise clinical relevant variations of the severity of esophagitis. The esophageal acid exposure data included in the validation of the LA classification system support the clinical relevance of this particular classification. Large prospective, randomised clinical trials have given the opportunity to evaluate further the clinical relevance of the LA classification. We found a significant correlation between the severity of heartburn and LA gradings. The subsequent clinical studies also found an impressive gradation of endoscopic healing relating to the pretreatment endoscopic grading [18-21]. The large number of patients involved in similar trials and the statistically significant differences are arguments for the clinical relevance of the LA grading system. Furthermore it is worth noting that the data obtained showed that the classification of patients into grade A and B seems to provide a clinical relevant subdivision both with regard to therapeutic response and also the subsequent course after cessation of therapy. These patients represent the most numerous groups of patients suffering from reflux disease that have previously been grouped somewhat ambiguously into one grade by for instance the Savary-Miller classification [14-17]. Symptom relapse curves separated patient who, before treatment, had an absence of esophageal mucosal breaks from those with LA grades A to C, respectively, indicating the relevance of similar information for the long-term management strategies of these patients [22-25].

It can therefore be concluded that the LA grading system identifies these lesions specific for GORD, gives an exact description of the lesion plus other findings, avoids overlap between grades and is easy to memorise. The LA grading system distinguishes between reversible and irreversible lesions and it has been scientifically validated which should offer unique opportunities for this system to become universally accepted.

References

1. Spechler SJ. Epidemiology and natural history of gastro-esophageal reflux disease. *Digestion* 1992; 51 (Suppl. 1): 24-9.
2. Bennett JR, Chapman RWG, Harvey RF, *et al.* Management guidelines for gastro-esophageal reflux disease. The European Digestive Disease Week, Amsterdam, 1991; 46-54.
3. Spechler SJ. Complications of gastro-esophageal reflux disease. In Castell DO, ed. *The esophagus*. Boston: Little Brown and Co, 1992: 543-56.
4. Dent J, Bremner CG, Collens MJ, *et al.* Barrett's esophagus. Working party report to the World Congress of Gastroenterology, Sydney 1990. *J Gastroenterol Hepatol* 1991; 6: 1-22.
5. Lundell L. Long-term treatment of gastro-esophageal reflux disease with omeprazole. *Scand J Gastroentrol* 1994; 29 (Suppl. 201): 74-8.
6. Armstrong D, Bennett JR, Blum AL, *et al.* The endoscopic assessment of esophagitis: a progress report on observer agreement. *Gastroenterology* 1996; 111: 85-92.
7. Lundell LR, Dent J, Blum MAL, Armstrong D, Galmiche JP, Johnson F, Hongo M, Richter JE, Spechler ST, Tytgat GNJ, Wallin L. Endoscopic assessment of esophagitis: clinical and functional correlates and further validation of the Los Angeles classification. *Gut* 1999; 45: 172-80.
8. Bytzer P, Havelund T, Möller Hansen J. Interobserver variation in the endoscopic diagnosis of reflux esophagitis. *Scand J Gastroenterol* 1993; 28: 119-25.
9. Cohen J. A coefficient of agreement for normal scales. *Educ Psychol Measurement* 1960; 20: 37-46.
10. Armstrong D, Emde C, Ianuen W, Blum AL. Diagnostic assessment of gastroesophageal reflux disease: what is possible vs what is practical? *Hepatogastroenterology* 1992; 39: 3-13.
11. Johnsson F, Weywadt L, Solhaug JH, *et al.* One week omeprazole treatment in the diagnosis of gastroesophageal reflux disease. *Scand J Gastroenterol* 1998; 33: 15-20.
12. Carlsson R. Gastroesophageal reflux disease (GERD) in primary care: an international study of different treatment strategies with omeprazole. *Eur J Gastroenterol Hepatol* 1998; 10: 119-24.
13. Carlsson R, Dent J, Bolling-Sternevald, *et al.* The usefulness of a structured questionnaire in the assessment of symptomatic gastroesophageal reflux disease. *Scand J Gastroenterol* 1998; 33: 1023-9.
14. Savary M, Miller G. *L'oesophage. Manuel et atlas d'endoscopie.* Soleure: Garsman Ab, 1977.
15. Monnier P, Savary M. Contribution of endoscopy to gastroesophageal reflux disease. *Scand J Gastroenterol* 1984; 106: 26.
16. Ollyo JB, Gontollier C, Bossard E, *et al.* La nouvelle classification de Savary des esophagitis de reflux. *Acta Endoscopica* 1992; 22: 307
17. Savary M. Miller G. *The esophagus. Handbook and atlas of endoscopy*. Solothorn, Switzerland: Gassman AG, 1978.
18. Ghillebert G, Demeyere AM, Jansson J, *et al.* How well can quantitative 24-hour intraesophageal pH monitoring distinguish various degrees of reflux disease? *Dig Dis Sci* 1995; 40: 1317-24.
19. Galmiche JP, Bruley des Varannes S. Symptoms and diseases severity in gastro-esophageal reflux disease. *Scand J Gastroenterol* 1994; 29: 62-8.
20. Pace F, Santalucia F, Bianchi Porro G. Natural History of gastro-esophageal reflux disease without esophagitis. *Gut* 1992; 32: 848-58.

21. Baldi F, Ferrarine F, Langanesi A, *et al*. Acid gastroesophageal reflux and symptom occurrence. Analyses of some factors influencing their association. *Dig Dis Sci* 1989; 34: 1890-3.
22. Hetzel DJ, Dent J, Reed WD, *et al*. Healing and relapse of severe peptic esophagitis after treatment with omeprazole. *Gastroenterology* 1988; 95: 901-12.
23. Sandmark S, Carlsson R, Fausa O, *et al*. Omeprazole or ranitidine in the treatment of reflux esophagitis. Results of double-blind, randomised, Scandinavian multicentre trial. *Scand J Gastroenterol* 1988; 23: 625-32.
24. Koelz HR, Birchler R, Bertholz A, *et al*. Healing and relapse or reflux esophagitis during treatment with ranitidine. *Gastroenterology* 1986; 91: 1198-205.
25. Dent J, Yeomans ND, Mackinnon M, *et al*. Omeprazole versus ranitidine for prevention of relapse in reflux esophagitis. A controlled double-blind trial of the efficacy and safety. *Gut* 1994; 35: 590-8.

An update on the pathogenesis of Barrett's esophagus

Prateek Sharma

University of Kansas School of Medicine, Veterans Affairs Medical Center, Kansas City, USA

Barrett's esophagus is the pre-malignant lesion for adenocarcinoma of the esophagus and the esophagogastric junction. It occurs on the background of chronic gastroesophageal reflux disease (GERD). The incidence of esophageal adenocarcinoma is rapidly rising; in fact it is the fastest rising incidence cancer in the Western world [1, 2]. This article will critically review the currently available data on the pathogenesis of Barrett's esophagus and adenocarcinoma. The role of acid and bile reflux in the development of Barrett's esophagus has been the subject of many animal and human studies.

Definition of Barrett's esophagus

The presence of columnar lining in the distal esophagus was first described by Norman Barrett, who described cases of esophageal ulcers surrounded by columnar mucosa (detected at autopsy). At that time, Barrett suggested that the ulcers developed in the stomach, which was displaced proximally [3]. Later in 1953, Allison and Johnstone published a paper describing in detail 7 cases of a columnar lined lower esophagus [4]. All these patients had erosive esophagitis and a hiatal hernia – suggesting that "Barrett's ulcers" might be a consequence of chronic gastroesophageal reflux. The definition and the concept of Barrett's esophagus have undergone a radical change since its first description in the 1950's to the present time where most of the data suggest that it is indeed an acquired disorder caused by reflux of gastroduodenal contents into the distal esophagus. The presence of a columnar lined distal esophagus of any length, with intestinal metaplasia on biopsy is the current definition of Barrett's esophagus [5].

Role of acid

A major advance in the understanding of the pathogenesis of Barrett's esophagus and the importance of gastroesophageal reflux (GER) is from the landmark study by Bremner *et al*. This experiment showed that regeneration of esophageal mucosa after severe mucosal injury from chronic GER in dogs occurred with columnar mucosa rather than squamous cells [6]. Other animal studies have also suggested that esophageal exposure to acid alone at higher concentrations or at lower concentrations in combination with pepsin results in esophageal mucosal injury predisposing to columnar metaplasia [7]. Another important observation was that patients having a distal esophagectomy with an esophagogastric anastomosis developed Barrett's esophagus just above the suture line [8]. The importance of acid in the pathogenesis of this lesion and this concept has been widely accepted since these earlier experimental studies and observations. The current hypothesis is that Barrett's mucosa develops from pluripotential stem cells, which are present in the basal layer of the esophageal mucosa [9]. There is no convincing evidence that patients with GERD and Barrett's secrete abnormally high gastric acid or pepsin compared to controls [10].

Clinical studies have confirmed the presence of severe GER in patients with Barrett's esophagus characterized by decreased lower esophageal sphincter (LES) pressure, delayed esophageal acid clearance, as well as increase in the frequency and duration of esophageal acid exposure [11, 12]. Patients with Barrett's esophagus have significantly higher exposure times to pH < 4 than healthy volunteers and even patients with GERD without Barrett's. Studies have also shown a positive correlation between the degree of abnormal acid exposure and the severity of esophagitis [12]. Compared to GERD patients without Barrett's, patients with Barrett's have on average lower LES pressure and the highest esophageal exposure times to acid on ambulatory pH monitoring [12, 13]. Esophageal acid exposure increases in patients with Barrett's esophagus compared to patients with GERD without erosive esophagitis. Also studies have supported the observation that the LES pressure in patients with Barrett's esophagus decreased to the same degree as seen with patients with severe esophagitis [13, 14]. In addition, patients with Barrett's esophagus have frequently associated hiatal hernias and ineffective peristalsis leading to defective clearance of the refluxed gastric contents [12, 14]. Recent studies have also shown the extent of columnar metaplasia to be related to the severity of gastroesophageal reflux and inversely to the LES pressure [15].

There is overwhelming clinical evidence supporting the association of GERD in Barrett's esophagus. At the time of upper endoscopy, Barrett's esophagus is detected in approximately 5-10% of patients with long-standing symptoms of reflux disease [16, 17]. There is a higher prevalence of hiatal hernia in patients with Barrett's esophagus. Cameron *et al*. reported the finding of a hiatal hernia in 96% of patients with long segment Barrett's esophagus (LSBE) and 72% of patients with short segment Barrett's esophagus (SSBE) [18]. The duration of reflux symptoms appears to be longer in patients with Barrett's than those without Barrett's esophagus. Hirota *et al*. reported the mean duration of reflux symptoms in patients with SSBE was 3.5 years, and was 20 years in those with LSBE [19]. Similarly, Lieberman *et al*. reported that patients with Barrett's esophagus had longer duration of symptoms as well as an early age of onset of GERD symptoms as opposed to GERD patients without Barrett's esophagus [20].

Barrett's esophagus seems to be an acquired lesion since the prevalence is very low in childhood, increases with age and is found in about 1% of adults over age 60 having endoscopy [17]. Further, the prevalence of Barrett's esophagus increases with age, particularly over age 50 [17], confirming that this lesion is acquired and not congenital and given its occurrence in patients with chronic GERD, it has now been postulated that it develops secondary to chronic GER.

Experimental and clinical evidence, thus, strongly supports the importance of acid and pepsin in causing esophageal mucosal injury.

Role of bile

The presence of Barrett's esophagus in patients with achlorhydria and post-gastrectomy states has suggested a possible role of duodenal contents in its pathogenesis. The duodenal content suspected of causing esophageal injury includes bile acids, lysolecithin and the pancreatic enzyme trypsin. Although commonly referred to as bile reflux, reflux of duodenal contents contains more than just bile, therefore the term duodenal gastroesophageal reflux (DGER) has been proposed.

On the other hand, the term alkaline reflux may be a misnomer and recent studies have questioned the accuracy of using just the pH as a marker for DGER [21, 22]; measurement of esophageal pH > 7 as a marker of DGER can be confounded by specific foods, oral disease, saliva, etc. A new fiber optic system (Bilitec) has been recently developed that detects bilirubin (as a marker of DGER) independent of the pH. Recent studies using this probe have reported a significant increase in both esophageal acid and bile exposure from controls to patients with esophagitis – the highest or the most abnormal values being in patients with Barrett's esophagus [23]. Reflux of acid parallels DGER, and both have been shown to be significantly higher in patients with Barrett's esophagus compared to controls and GERD patients without Barrett's esophagus [23, 24].

Thus, current studies reveal that both gastric and duodenal contents mix together and reflux into the esophagus in an acid environment. However, the individual contributions and influences of acid, pepsin, bile and other duodenal contents in patients with Barrett's esophagus remain to be determined. The degree and the extent of GER and DGER parallels the severity of GERD – increasing from healthy controls to patients with Barrett's esophagus. These findings suggest a synergism between acid, pepsin and conjugated bile acids that contribute to the development of Barrett's esophagus and subsequently to dysplasia and adenocarcinoma.

Role of salivary and esophageal secretions

Patients with Barrett's esophagus have been shown to have impaired secretory function of salivary glands – the content of salivary glycoconjugates and epidermal growth factor (EGF). This may be of clinical importance since EGF is responsible for inhibition of hydrogen ion diffusion. Also, patients with Barrett's esophagus exhibit impairment in esophageal EGF secretion [25]. Such abnormalities of salivary and esophageal glandular function could compromise the protective function of the esophageal mucous lining, rendering the exposed mucosa susceptible to injury caused by esophageal acid reflux or resulting in a failure of mucosal repair.

Demographics

Barrett's esophagus is primarily detected in Caucasians; the reason for this pre-dominance is not clear. Even in a large African American population in South Africa, only 5% of the Barrett's esophagus cohorts were African American [26]. Barrett's esophagus and adenocarcinoma are rare in the Asian population – comparable to the low incidence in the United States before the 1970's. Barrett's esophagus also seems to be uncommon outside of North America, Europe and Australia. It is detected in 0.1-0.3% of upper endoscopies in Japan (as opposed to 1% in the United States) and this difference between Eastern and Western populations may be due to differences in the prevalence of GERD [27]. For example, in Singapore the prevalence of heartburn in adults is 1.6% (on a monthly basis) compared to 29-44% in the Western countries [28]. The mean age of diagnosis of Barrett's is in the 60's at which time the patient may have had unrecognized Barrett's for many years [17].

The prevalence of Barrett's esophagus for unknown reasons is higher in males than in females. This has been reported from both European as well as US studies. The ratio has been reported to vary from 2-3:1 for males to females [29]. However, the similar ratio for esophageal adenocarcinoma, also high in males, is much greater, *i.e.* 8:1 (male: female). Thus, Barrett's esophagus appears to be more prevalent in Caucasians, in males as well as in the more developed countries.

Studies have demonstrated that the average length of Barrett's esophagus is identical when patients are separated by age [29] and that no change in the overall length of Barrett's esophagus is observed on follow-up [30] – indicating that susceptible individuals have developed their entire length at the time of recognition.

Barrett's esophagus has rarely been reported in children. From the Mayo Clinic data, only one in 679 patients between the ages 10-19 years was diagnosed with Barrett's esophagus and none below age 10 had Barrett's esophagus [17]. Hassal, *et al.* reported the youngest proven case at age 7 and even this childhood condition was acquired and associated with GERD [31].

Role of genetic factors

Studies have shown that relatives of patients with Barrett's esophagus and also relatives of patients with esophageal adenocarcinoma have reflux symptoms 2-3 times more commonly than controls [32]. These findings suggest that there may be an inherited predisposition to reflux disease. Reports are available of families in which 2 or more members of Barrett's esophagus are involved in one generation [33, 34].

Role of *Helicobacter pylori*

The incidence of GERD and esophageal adenocarcinoma has increased in recent years, whereas the incidence of *H. pylori* associated peptic ulcer disease and distal gastric adenocarcinomas has declined [35]. This suggests an inverse relationship between *H. pylori* infection and esophageal disease. While *H. pylori* infection clearly does not cause GERD, it may protect certain susceptible individuals from the development of GERD and its complications.

Recent studies suggest that infection with *H. pylori*, especially cagA strains, may protect against the development of Barrett's esophagus dysplasia and adenocarcinoma. In a study of 210 patients with GERD and Barrett's, Vicari *et al.* found a lower prevalence of *H. pylori* infection (34%) in patients with Barrett's esophagus compared to an age match control group (46%) but this was not a significant difference [36]. However, when compared to controls (42%), the prevalence of cagA *H. pylori* was significantly decreased in patients with Barrett's esophagus (13.3%) and Barrett's with adenocarcinoma/dysplasia (0%). These findings indicate that cagA *H.pylori* may potentially protect against complications of GERD such as Barrett's and associated dysplasia/adenocarcinoma. Similarly, Chow *et al.* reported that the carriage of cagA strain was associated with an increased risk for distal gastric cancer but reduced risk for esophageal and gastric cardia adenocarcinoma [37].

Emerging evidence also suggests that severity of corpus gastritis may protect against the development of GERD [38]. Gastric acid hypo-secretion has been described in a subgroup of *H. pylori* infected patients, specifically those with corpus pre-dominant gastritis and increased gastric atrophy. Therefore, the distribution and severity of gastritis caused by H. *pylori* infection rather than simply the presence or absence of the organism may be an important factor in the development of GERD, Barrett's esophagus and esophageal adenocarcinoma.

Increasing incidence of esophageal adenocarcinoma

Patients with Barrett's esophagus have a 30-125 time increased risk of developing esophageal adenocarcinoma compared to the general population. Recent studies from the United States have suggested an incidence of cancer of about 1 in 200 patient-years of follow-up [39]. Studies from the UK suggest a much higher incidence of esophageal adenocarcinoma. Esophageal adenocarcinomas now account for over 50% of esophageal cancers in many reports. Population based studies from the United States and Western Europe have shown a dramatic increase in the incidence of adenocarcinoma starting in the 1970's to the early 1990's [1, 2]. The exact etiologies for this rising incidence is unclear and whether there has been a true increase in Barrett's esophagus also remains controversial.

Reports from Olmstead County indicate an increase in the number of clinically diagnosed Barrett's esophagus patients from 3.7/100,000 in the 1960's to 10.5/100,000 in the late 1990's. However, at the same time, the number of upper endoscopic examinations performed has also increased in a similar fashion. These data suggest that this increase may be secondary to an increased detection rather than a true increase [29]. However, in Scotland, they have detected an increase in cases from 0.14/100 endoscopies in the 1980's to 4.27/100 endoscopies in early 1990's [40]. Another small study has reported that the prevalence of long segment Barrett's esophagus has remained unchanged, however, the prevalence of short segment Barrett's esophagus has increased, even after taking into account the number of endoscopies [41].

In an attempt to better explain the rapidly rising incidence of esophageal adenocarcinoma, attention has recently been focused on its epidemiology. Increasing obesity in the Western world along with an increase in GERD have been proposed as mechanisms for the increasing incidence of esophageal adenocarcinoma. A protective effect of *Helicobacter pylori* has been suggested as an alternative hypothesis. Gammon *et al.* reported that the odds ratio for current smoking was 2.2 times greater and for ex-smokers was 2.0 times greater in the cancer cases compared to controls [42]. The authors concluded that smoking could account for 40% of adenocarcinomas and the increased risk persisted up to 30 years after quitting smoking. Chow *et al.* found that the body mass index (BMI) was related to increasing esophageal adenocarcinoma [43]. The odds ratio for obesity was 2.9 times greater in the heaviest 25% of the population compared to the lightest. These authors concluded that obesity would account for 33% of adenocarcinomas. These factors associated with esophageal adenocarcinoma may also be linked to the development of Barrett's esophagus; however the pathogenesis of Barrett's esophagus has not been well explored.

Conclusion

Both genetic and environmental factors including acid reflux and duodenal gastroesophageal reflux are involved in the pathogenesis of Barrett's esophagus and esophageal adenocarcinoma *(figure 1)*. Symptoms of gastroesophageal reflux disease are highly prevalent in the adult white population, however, Barrett's esophagus develops in the minority of these patients and most of these patients will not develop adenocarcinoma during their lifetime. The increasing incidence of esophageal adenocarcinoma has raised concerns in both patients and physicians alike, especially given its direct link to GERD. Changes in diet, increasing obesity, drugs, tobacco use and decreasing prevalence *H. pylori* have been linked to this rising incidence.

Barrett's esophagus occurs as a result of increased esophageal acid exposure. Abnormalities, similar to those in patients with erosive esophagitis, including a compromised anti-reflux barrier, prolonged esophageal acid clearance, and presence of hiatal hernia are consistently found in patients with Barrett's esophagus. It has been shown in both animal and human studies that acid is a key agent in causing esophageal mucosal injury. This

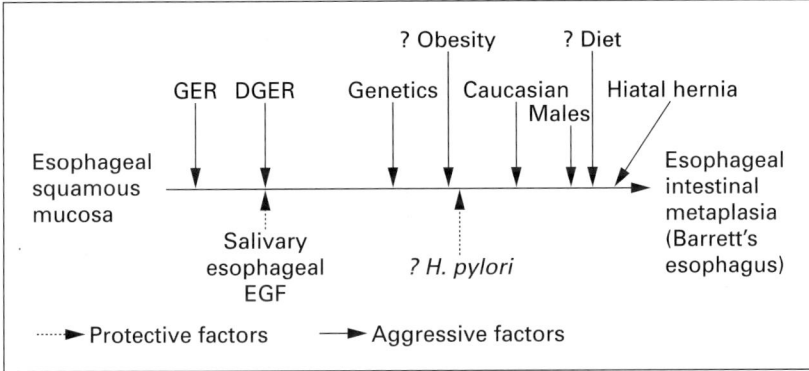

Figure 1. Factors associated in the pathogenesis of Barrett's esophagus.

observation has been supplemented by recent data that DGER occurs along with reflux of gastric acid. The degree of esophageal acid and bile exposure is more marked in patients with Barrett's esophagus, thus raising the possibility that synergism exists between acid pepsin, and conjugated bile acids. Why some patients with GERD develop Barrett's and others doesn't suggest a genetic predisposition.

Future

Identification of a simple marker or markers that would allow stratification of patients that are at high risk for development of Barrett's esophagus would be very useful. This can potentially eliminate the need for endoscopy for all patients with GERD and help focus resources on a subset of high risk patients. Validation of a simple blood test, unsedated small caliber upper endoscopy or other non-endoscopic techniques (like balloon cytology, colorimetric recognition) hold promise for the future.

References

1. Devesa SS, Blot WJ, Fraumeni JF. Changing patterns in the incidence of esophageal and gastric carcinoma in the United States. *Cancer* 1998; 83: 2049-53.
2. Blot WJ, Devesa SS, Fraumeni JF Jr. Continuing climb in rates of esophageal adenocarcinoma: an update. *JAMA* 1993; 270: 1320 (letter).
3. Barrett NR. Chronic peptic ulcer of the oesophagus and "esophagitis". *Br J Surg* 1950; 38: 175-82.
4. Allison PR, Johnstone AS. Esophagus lined with gastric mucous membrane. *Thorax* 1953; 8: 87-93.
5. Weinstein WM, Ippoliti AF. The diagnosis of Barrett's esophagus: Goblets, goblets, goblets. *Gastrointest Endosc* 1996; 44: 91-5.
6. Bremner CG, Lynch VP, Ellis FH. Barrett's esophagus: congenital or acquired? An experimental study of esophageal mucosal regeneration in the dog. *Surgery* 1970; 68: 209-16.
7. Goldberg HI, Dodds WJ, Gee S, Montgomery C, Zboralske FF. Role of acid and pepsin in acute experimental esophagitis. *Gastroenterology* 1969; 56: 223-30.

8. Hamilton SR, Yardley JH. Regeneration of cardiac type mucosa and acquisition of Barrett's mucosa after esophagogastrostomy. *Gastroenterology* 1977; 72: 669-75.
9. Gillen P, Keeling P, Byrne PJ, *et al.* Experimental columnar metaplasia in the canine oesophagus. *Br J Surg* 1988; 75: 113-5.
10. Hirschowitz BI. Gastric acid and pepsin secretion in patients with Barrett's esophagus and appropriate controls. *Dig Dis Sci* 1996; 41: 1384-91.
11. Stein HJ, Hoeft S, DeMeester TR. Functional foregut abnormalities in Barrett's esophagus. *J Thorac Cardiovasc Surg* 1993; 105: 107-11.
12. Iascone C, DeMeester TR, Little AG, *et al.* Functional assessment, proposed pathogenesis and surgical therapy. *Arch Surg* 1983; 118: 543-9.
13. Coenraad M, Masclee AA, Straathof JW, Ganesh S, Griffioen G, Lamers CB. Is Barrett's esophagus characterized by more pronounced acid reflux than severe esophagitis? *Am J Gastroenterol* 1998; 93(7): 1068-72.
14. Parrilla P, Ortiz A, Martinez DE, Haro LF, *et al.* Evaluation of the magnitude of gastro-oesophageal reflux in Barrett's esophagus. *Gut* 1990; 31: 964-7.
15. Oberg S, DeMeester TR, Peters JH, Hagen JA, *et al.* The extent of Barrett's esophagus depends on the status of the lower esophageal sphincter and the degree of esophageal acid exposure. *J Thorac Cardiovasc Surg* 1999; 117: 572-80.
16. Winters C, Spurling TJ, Chobanian SJ, Curtis DJ, Esposito RL, Hacker JF, Johnson DA, Cruess DF, Cotelingam JD, Gurney MS, Cattau EL. Barrett's esophagus. A prevalent, occult complication of gastroesophageal reflux disease. *Gastroenterology* 1987; 92: 118-24.
17. Cameron AJ, Lomboy CT. Barrett's esophagus; age, prevalence and the extent of columnar epithelium. *Gastroenterology* 1992; 103: 1241-5.
18. Cameron AJ. Barrett's esophagus: prevalence and size of hiatal hernia. *Am J Gastroenterol* 1999; 94 (8): 2054-9.
19. Hirota WK, Loughney TM, Lazas DJ, Maydonovitch CL, Rholl V, Wong RKH. Specialized intestinal metaplasia dysplasia and cancer of the esophagus and esophagogastric junction: prevalence and clinical data. *Gastroenterology* 1999; 116: 277-85.
20. Lieberman DA, Oehlke M, Helfand M, and the GORGE consortium. Risk factors for Barrett's esophagus in community-based practice. *Am J Gastroenterol* 1997; 92: 1293-7.
21. Singh S, Bradley LA, Richter JE. Determinants of oesophageal "alkaline" pH environment in controls and patients with gastro-oesophageal reflux disease. *Gut* 1993; 34: 309-16.
22. DeVault KR, Georgeson S, Castell DO. Salivary stimulation mimics esophageal exposure to refluxed duodenal contents. *Am J Gastroenterol* 1993; 88: 1040-3.
23. Vaezi MF, Richter JE. Role of acid and duodenogastroesophageal reflux in gastroesophageal reflux disease. *Gastroenterology* 1996; 111: 1192-9.
24. Marshall REK, Anggiansah A, Owen WA, Owen WJ. The relationship between acid and bile reflux and symptoms of gastro-oesophageal reflux disease. *Gut* 1997; 40: 182-7.
25. Rourk RM, Namiot Z, Sarosiek J, *et al.* Diminished content of esophageal epidermal growth factor in patients with reflux esophagitis. *Am J Gastroenterol* 1994; 89: 1177-84.
26. Mason RJ, Bremner CG. The columnar-lined (Barrett's) oesophagus in black patients. *S Afr J Surg* 1998; 36: 61-2.
27. Shoji T, Hongo M, Fukudo S, Handa M, Inaba H, Kano M, Narita H, Tamura D. Increasing incidence of Barrett's esophagus and Barrett's carcinoma in Japan. *Gastroenterology* 1999; 116: A312.
28. Ho KY, Kang JY, Seow A. Prevalence of gastrointestinal symptoms in a multiracial Asian population, with particular reference to reflux-type symptoms. *Am J Gastroenterol* 1998; 93: 1816-22.
29. Cameron AJ. Epidemiology of columnar-lined esophagus and adenocarcinoma. *Gastrenterolo Clin North Am* 1997; 26: 484-7.

30. Sharma P, Sampliner RE, Camargo E. Normalization of esophageal pH with high dose proton pump inhibitory therapy does not result in regression of Barrett's esophagus. *Am J Gastroenterol* 1997; 92: 582-5.
31. Hassell E. Barrett's esophagus: congenital or acquired? *Am J Gastroenterol* 1993; 88: 819-24.
32. Romero Y, Cameron AJ, Locke GR III, *et al.* Familial aggregation of gastroesophageal reflux in patients with Barrett's esophagus and esophageal adenocarcinoma. *Gastroenterology* 1997; 113: 1449-56.
33. Jochem VJ, Fuerst PA, Fromkes JJ. Familial Barrett's esophagus associated with adenocarcinoma. *Gastroenterology* 1992; 102: 1400-12.
34. Fahmy N, King JF. Barrett's esophagus: an acquired condition with genetic predisposition. *Am J Gastroenterol* 1993; 88: 1262-5.
35. El-Serag HB, Sonnenberg A. Opposing time trends of peptic ulcer and reflux disease. *Gut* 1998; 43: 327-33.
36. Vicari JJ, Peck RM, Falk GW, *et al.* The seroprevalence of *cagA* positive *Helicobacter pylori* strains in the spectrum of gastroesophageal reflux disease. *Gastroenterology* 1998; 115: 50-7.
37. Chow WH, Blaser MJ, Blot WJ, *et al.* An inverse relation between $cagA^+$ strains of *Helicobacter pylori* infection and risk of esophageal and gastric cardia adenocarcinoma. *Cancer Res* 1998; 58: 588-90.
38. Labenz J, Blum AL, Bayerdorffer E, *et al.* Curing *Helicobacter pylori* infection in patients with duodenal ulcer disease may provoke reflux esophagitis. *Gastroenterology* 1997; 112: 1442-7.
39. Drewitz DJ, Sampliner RE, Garewal HS. The incidence of adenocarcinoma in Barrett's esophagus: A prospective study of 170 patients followed 4.8 years. *Am J Gastroenterol* 1997; 92: 212-5.
40. Prach AJ, MacDonald TA, Hopwood DA, Johnston DA. Increasing incidence of Barrett's oesophagus: education, enthusiasm or epidemiology? *Lancet* 1997; 350: 933.
41. Sharma P, Sampliner RE. Increasing incidence of adenocarcinoma of the esophagus (EA) and esophagogastric junction (EGJA) – is short segment Barrett's esophagus (SSBE) responsible? *Am J Gastroenterol* 1998; 93: 1624.
42. Gammon MD, Schoenberg JB, Ahsan H, *et al.* Tobacco, alcohol and socioeconomic status and adenocarcinoma of the esophagus and gastric cardia. *J Natl Cancer Inst* 1997; 89: 1277-84.
43. Chow WH, Blot WJ, Vaughan WJ, *et al.* Body mass index and risk of adenocarcinomas of the esophagus and gastric cardia. *J Natl Cancer Inst* 1998; 9 (0): 150-5.

Surveillance of Barrett's esophagus: to screen or not to screen?

Guido N.J. Tytgat

*Academic Medical Center, Department of Gastroenterology and Hepatology,
Amsterdam Zuidoost, The Netherlands*

Esophageal columnar metaplasia or intestinal metaplasia or so-called Barrett's esophagus is an established precursor of esophageal and gastroesophageal junction adenocarcinoma. Barrett's esophagus patients are usually considered to have a 30-125 times increased risk of developing esophageal adenocarcinoma [1-3]. The incidence of Barrett's adenocarcinoma derived from prospective studies varies from one in 52 to one in 208 patient-years [4-10]. Yet recent studies would indicate that this risk is overrated due to publication bias [11].

Pathogenesis

The mechanisms that lead to esophageal columnar metaplasia and dysplasia are poorly understood. Although we know that patients with columnar metaplasia usually have rather severe gastroesophageal acid reflux and often also have a component of duodeno-gastro-esophageal (biliary) reflux and almost always have a rather large hiatal hernia responsible for a common cavity phenomenon, in practice it remains very difficult to predict which patients with reflux disease will ultimately develop columnar metaplasia [12].

It is also largely unknown at which time columnar metaplasia develops. Most often patients are discovered as having columnar metaplasia beyond 50 years of age and it is impossible at that time to appreciate when the columnar metaplasia has developed and/or whether the metaplasia is progressive.

Once Barrett's has been diagnosed, endoscopic biopsy surveillance is usually recommended for the detection of either high-grade dysplasia or adenocarcinoma at an early, curable stage [13-17]. Which patients are at risk of developing dysplastic changes and the velocity of such developments remains beyond our current understanding. Also the progression of dysplasia from low to high grade and ultimately to cancer proves to be highly variable from one person to the other. Two studies have looked at that problem more in detail, a European and an American study *(figure 1* and *figure 2)* [18, 19]. The velocity of progressive worsening of dysplasia to ultimately early cancer is highly different from patient to patient. Because it is impossible at present to predict when and how rapidly metaplasia and dysplasia develop, one has to rely on a standardized mucosal sampling protocol. Currently most clinicians certainly in the Western world do follow the guidelines designed by the American College of Gastroenterology [20]. In essence the advice is to carry out a surveillance endoscopy with four quadrant biopsies every two cm every three or perhaps every five years when there is no evidence of dysplastic change. If some of the biopsies do reveal low grade dysplasia, the advice is to repeat the endoscopy every six months for the first year, and if there is no further worsening, then to continue surveillance annually. It is somewhat unclear what to do if further biopsies do not reveal dysplastic change. Empirically some would consider the patient at low risk, if there are two further endoscopies without any evidence of dysplasia. In case biopsies do reveal high grade dysplasia,

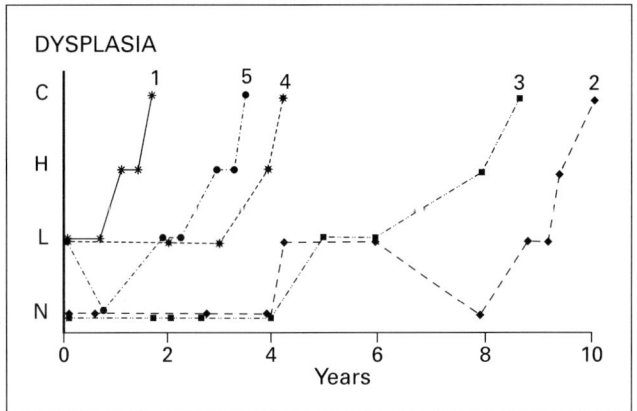

Figure 1. Development and progression of dysplasia in 5 patients with Barrett's esophagus who developed carcinoma. N: negative for dysplasia; L: low-grade dysplasia (including indefinite for dysplasia): H: high-grade dysplasia; C: carcinoma.

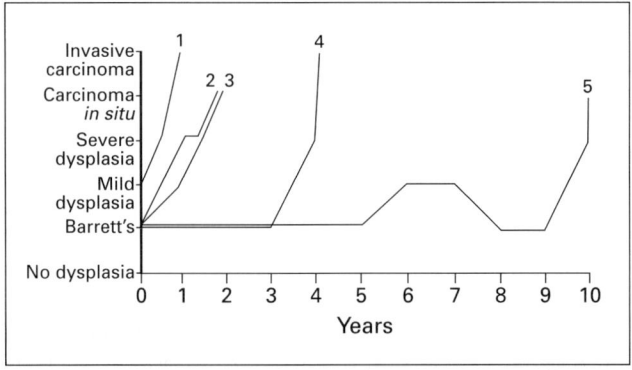

Figure 2. The progression of dysplasia to carcinoma in five patients with Barrett's esophagus.

the advice is to repeat the biopsies some three months later after intense medical therapy and to have the biopsies checked by another experienced histopathologist. Obviously at that time it is also mandatory to rule out early cancer. Preferably this should be done by endosonography using high frequency ultrasound.

Once high grade dysplasia is discovered, esophageal resection should be discussed if the patient is a good surgical risk. If esophageal resection is contra-indicated, then ablative therapy should be considered such as mucosal resection of the dysplastic area [21], followed either by additional mucosectomy of the surrounding mucosa or photodynamic therapy or other ablative therapies.

Although endoscopic bioptic surveillance of Barrett's esophagus is recommended [22, 23], the exact interval in routine practice remains controversial and highly variable from unspecified to as frequent as every 12 months, up to every 5 years [2, 6, 14, 24-28]. Identification of simple, easily attainable, noncumbersome clinical, endoscopic, and histological features that could accurately predict the development of Barrett's adenocarcinoma (*i.e.*, risk stratification) and hence provide a guide for timing of surveillance examinations, would be of tremendous utility in this era of medical cost containment.

To what extent the current guidelines are followed in clinical practice is largely unknown [29]. Even when followed adequately it is not known whether this methodology allows accurate detection of columnar metaplasia/dysplasia development. Several critical statements have been voiced in the literature, casting doubt on the validity of such screening policy. Yet, despite such inherent weaknesses standardized mucosal sampling remains for the time being the only possible method to detect worsening dysplasia.

Impact of endoscopic biopsy surveillance of Barrett's esophagus on pathological stage and clinical outcome of Barrett's carcinoma

Symptoms of esophageal cancer generally correspond with the stage of the disease. Patients who initially present with dysphagia often have a dismal prognosis after surgery as obstructive symptoms usually indicate the presence of advanced disease [30]. On the other hand, patients who undergo surgery for Barrett's carcinoma that is limited to the mucosa or submucosa (T1-tumor), have a favorable prognosis, with a 60%-100% 5-year survival [31-33]. Since early adenocarcinomas in Barrett's esophagus give only rarely symptoms, detection of cancer at an early, curable stage can only be achieved by surveillance. The relatively high risk of carcinoma together with the poor prognosis of a symptomatic cancer seems sufficient to warrant a surveillance program for patients with a Barrett's esophagus. Although its cost-effectiveness has been questioned by some authors [34, 35], two recent studies indicate that the cost of endoscopic surveillance to detect adenocarcinoma in Barrett's esophagus compares favourably with the cost of screening mammography to detect early breast cancer [36, 37]. The major concern is a lack of evidence that surveillance of Barrett's esophagus reduces mortality from esophageal cancer. The ideal methodology for the evaluation of the efficacy of surveillance programs is the randomized trial. Such a trial not only seems impractical in terms of the number of patients needed and the many years of follow-up [38], it may also pose an ethical dilemma for the physician who is to withhold a potentially life-saving procedure from the individual patient with a premalignant condition. Therefore, it is unlikely that a randomized study will ever be performed for cancer surveillance in Barrett's esophagus. The ongoing discussion will have to rely upon more or less indirect evaluation of its effect on cancer mortality rate.

The study by Van Sandick *et al.* [39] suggests that endoscopic biopsy surveillance provides a beneficial effect on resectability and mortality from cancer in Barrett's esophagus. In parallel with the findings of other authors [36, 27, 40] patients who had undergone some form of endoscopic surveillance were operated on at significantly earlier stages of their disease, with a subsequent survival advantage over patients who had not been part of a surveillance program. Comparing the outcome of surveillance-detected cases with that of symptom-diagnosed cases, is probably the most commonly used method. Nonrandomized types of evaluation harbor a number of pitfalls [41, 42]. First, one must be aware of selection bias. Patients undergoing regular surveillance tend to be health-conscious and may be the ones who would have presented with early-stage cancers even if their disease was diagnosed because of symptoms. Secondly, lead time bias operates in all screening and surveillance programs [43]. An observed survival benefit may be due only to the advancement of the diagnosis of cancer in time, and not to the postponement of death. Finally, the evaluation of cancer screening is subject to length bias [44]. This occurs because screening programs are more likely to detect slow-growing lesions with a good prognosis than lesions with a more aggressive nature and relatively unfavorable prognosis. Importantly, the stage distribution and duration of survival in the surveillance-group may partly reflect the lead time and length bias for cancer in Barrett's esophagus. To acknowledge these factors, results should be analyzed on an 'intention to surveillance' basis. In search for dysplastic foci, the entire length of the Barrett's mucosa should be sampled. It can be expected that in clinical practice surveillance programs will be less than perfect. In a majority of patients, the development of invasive adenocarcinoma was preceded by detection of dysplastic epithelium. Although "regression" of low-grade dysplasia is said to be possible, the subsequent development of adenocarcinoma or high-grade dysplasia suggests that this observation is probably due to sampling error or histopathological misinterpretation.

When high-grade dysplasia is found, a clinical dilemma is often encountered. In centers with a low operative mortality, high-grade dysplasia is increasingly regarded as the end point of surveillance for patients in whom a major operation is feasible [45-49]. Other authors reserve esophagectomy for proven invasive adenocarcinoma and propose continued surveillance for high-grade dysplasia by strict endoscopic biopsy protocols [50-52]. Importantly, high-grade dysplasia has not only been identified as a predictor of future cancer development, it may also indicate the presence of a coexisting invasive adenocarcinoma. A recent collective series of 96 patients who underwent esophagectomy for high-grade dysplasia showed a 41% incidence of endoscopically undetected adenocarcinoma. This finding emphasizes the limitation of at random biopsies in detecting foci of malignancy in Barrett's esophagus. Endoscopic biopsy surveillance of patients with Barrett's esophagus permits detection of cancer at an early, curable stage. In contrast, the majority of patients who initally presented with Barrett's carcinoma did not survive the first two years after operative treatment.

Discussion

Numerous studies have clearly demonstrated that the histological progression of Barrett's to adenocarcinoma involves a progressive, stepwise sequence of events characterized by the successive appearance of Barrett's metaplasia negative for dysplasia, low grade dysplasia / indefinite dysplasia, high grade dysplasia, and eventually adenocarcinoma. The presence of high grade dysplasia as a marker for progression to adenocarcinoma has already been well established [4, 6, 9, 53-57] and is itself an indication for esophagectomy according to many authorities [52, 58, 59]. The incidence of progression to adenocarcinoma in patients with high grade dysplasia prospectively followed has been reported to range from 17% to 66% [9, 55, 60-63], in a time interval ranging from 0.75 - 9 years. The risk of low grade dysplasia / indefinite dysplasia progression to adenocarcinoma is not as well characterized as that for high grade dysplasia. Progression of low grade dysplasia / indefinite dysplasia at index diagnosis to either multifocal high grade dysplasia [50] or cancer [50] is possible. However, the vast majority of patients with index low grade dysplasia / indefinite dysplasia eventually regress to no dysplasia. Identification of additional markers, such as p53 tumor suppressor gene mutation or flow cytometric abnormalities of aneuploidy and/or increased G2/tetraploid populations [63], as a means to identify which patients with index low grade dysplasia / indefinite dysplasia are at risk for progression, would be extremely helpful to further delineate surveillance intervals for this subgroup of patients.

Length of Barrett's esophagus was identified by Iftikhar *et al.* [10] as an important factor in the development of Barrett's dysplasia and adenocarcinoma. However, it has been well established that dysplasia and adenocarcinoma can occur in Barrett's mucosa of all lengths [62]. Overall however the prevalence of dysplasia and adenocarcinoma, as well as the incidence of dysplasia, is significantly less in patients with short segment Barrett [64].

The presence of medium- or large-sized hiatal hernia as a risk factor for the development of Barrett's cancer needs further substantiation. Theoretically the larger the hiatal hernia, the greater the disruption of the antireflux barrier, the greater the likelihood of pathological reflux, and the more severe the reflux injury to the esophageal mucosa, which may ultimately provide a stronger stimulus for neoplastic progression. Most important at the present are the endoscopic features (length of Barrett's segment and hiatal hernia) and especially the histology (dysplasia at initial diagnosis or during follow-up) which are predictive of development of multifocal high grade dysplasia/adenocarcinoma.

References

1. Spechler SJ, Robbins AH, Rubins HB, *et al.* Adenocarcinoma and Barrett's esophagus. An overrated risk? *Gastroenterology* 1984; 87: 927-33.
2. Cameron AJ, Ott BJ, Payne WS. The incidence of adenocarcinoma in columnar-lined (Barrett's) esophagus. *N Engl J Med* 1985; 313: 857-8.
3. Williamson WA, Ellis FH, Gibb SP, *et al.* Barrett's esophagus. Prevalence and incidence of adenocarcinoma. *Arch Intern Med* 1991; 151: 2212-6.

4. Hameeteman W, Tytgat GNJ, Houthoff HJ, et al. Barrett's esophagus: Development of dysplasia and adenocarcinoma. *Gastroenterology* 1989; 96: 1249-56.
5. Dent J, Bremner CG, Collen MJ, et al. Barrett's esophagus: Working Party Report to World Congresses of Gastroenterology, Sydney, 1990. *J Gastroenterol Hepatol* 1991; 6: 1-22.
6. Robertson CS, Mayberry JF, Nicholson DA, et al. Value of endoscopic surveillance in the detection of neoplastic change in Barrett's esophagus. *Br J Surg* 1988; 75: 760-3.
7. Drewitz DJ, Sampliner RE, Garewal HS: The incidence of adenocarcinoma in Barrett's esophagus: A prospective study of 170 patients followed 4.8 years. *Am J Gastroenterol* 1997; 92: 212-5.
8. Bonelli L, GOSPE: Barrett's esophagus: Results of a multicentric survey. *Endoscopy* 1993; 25 (suppl): 652-4.
9. Miros M, Kerlin P, Walker N. Only patients with dysplasia progress to adenocarcinoma in Barrett's esophagus. *Gut* 1991; 32: 1441-6.
10. Iftikhar SY, James PD, Stelle RJC, et al. Length of Barrett's esophagus: An important factor in the development of dysplasia and adenocarcinoma. *Gut* 1992; 33: 1155-8.
11. Shaheen NJ, Crosby MA, Bozymski EM, Sandler RS. Is there publication bias in the reporting of cancer risk in Barrett's esophagus? *Gastroenterology* 2000; 119: 333-8.
12. Weston AP, Badr AS, Hassanein RS. Prospective multivariate analysis of clinical, endoscopic, and histological factors predictive of the development of Barrett's multifocal high-grade dysplasia or adenocarcinoma. *Am J Gastroenterol* 94: 3413-9.
13. Spechler SJ: Endoscopic surveillance for patients with Barrett's esophagus: Does the cancer risk justify the practice? *Ann Intern Med* 1987; 106: 902-4.
14. Riddell RH: Early detection of neoplasia of the esophagus and gastroesophageal junction. *Am J Gastroenterol* 1996; 91: 853-63.
15. Richter JE. Endoscopic surveillance of Barrett's esophagus: Another viewpoint. *Am J Gastroenterol* 1993; 88: 630-2.
16. Spechler SJ. Barrett's esophagus. *Semin Oncol* 1994; 21: 431-7.
17. Spechler SJ, Goyal RK: Cancer surveillance in Barrett's esophagus: What is the endpoint? *Gastroenterology* 1994; 106: 275-6.
18. Hameeteman W, Tytgat GNJ, Houthoff HJ, Van Den Tweel JG: Barrett's esophagus: development of dysplasia and adenocarcinoma. *Gastroenterology* 1989; 96: 249-56.
19. Williamson WA, Ellis FH, Gibb SP, Shahian DM, Aretz HT, Heatley GJ, Watkins E. Barrett's Esophagus. Prevalence and Incidence of Adenocarcinoma. *Arch Intern Med* 1991; 151: 2212-6.
20. Sampliner RE, and The Practice Parameters Committee of the American College of Gastroenterology. Practice Guidelines on the Diagnosis, Surveillance, and Therapy of Barrett's Esophagus. *Am J Gastroenterol* 1998; 93: 1028-32.
21. Ell C, May A, Gossner L, Pech O, Günter E et al. Endoscopic mucosal resection of early cancer and high-grade dysplasia in Barrett's esophagus. *Gastroenterology* 2000; 118: 670-7.
22. Policy and procedure manual for GI endoscopy: Guidelines for training and practice. Manchester, MA: *American Society for GI Endoscopy*, 1990.
23. American Society for GI Endoscopy. The role of endoscopy in the surveillance of premalignant conditions of the upper GI tract. Guidelines for clinical application. *Gastrointest Endosc* 1988; 34: 18S-20S.
24. Reid BJ. Barrett's esophagus and esophageal adenocarcinoma. *Gastroenterol Clin North Am* 1991; 20: 817-34.
25. Streitz JM Jr, Williamson WA, Ellis FH Jr. Current concepts concerning the nature and treatment of Barrett's esophagus and its complications. *Ann Thorac Surg* 1992; 54: 586-91.
26. Kruse P, Boesby S, Bernstein IT, et al. Barrett's esophagus and esophageal adenocarcinoma. Endoscopic and histological surveillance. *Scand J Gastroenterol* 1993; 28: 193-6.
27. Streitz JM Jr, Andrews CW Jr, Ellis FH Jr. Endoscopic surveillance of Barrett's esophagus. Does it help? *J Thorac Cardiovasc Surg* 1993; 105: 383-8.

28. Provenzale D, Kep JA, Arora S, et al. A guide for surveillance of patients with Barrett's esophagus. *Am J Gastroenterol* 1994; 89: 670-80.
29. Van Sandick JW, Bartelsman JFWM, Van Lanschot JJB, Tytgat GNJ, Obertop H. Surveillance of Barrett esophagus: physicians' practices and review of current guidelines. *Eur J Gastroenterol Hepatol* 2000; 12: 111-7.
30. Streitz JM Jr, Ellis FH Jr, Gibb SP, et al. Adenocarcinoma in Barrett's esophagus. A clinicopathologic study of 65 cases. *Ann Surg* 1991; 213: 122-5.
31. DeMeester TR, Attwood SEA, Smyrk TC, et al. Surgical therapy in Barrett's esophagus. *Ann Surg* 1990; 212: 528-40.
32. Menke-Pluymers MBE, Schoute NW, Mulder AH, et al. Outcome of surgical treatment of adenocarcinoma in Barrett's esophagus. *Gut* 1992; 33: 1454-8.
33. Lerut T, Coosemans W, Van Raemdonk D, et al. Surgical treatment of Barrett's carcinoma. Correlations between morphologic findings and prognosis. *J Thorac Cardiovasc Surg* 1994; 107: 1059-65.
34. Lederle FA. Endoscopic surveillance of patients with Barrett's esophagus. *Ann Intern Med* 1987; 107: 592-3.
35. Van Der Burgh A, Dees J, Hop WCJ, Van Blankenstein M. Esophageal cancer is an uncommon cause of death in patients with Barrett's esophagus. *Gut* 1996; 39: 5-8.
36. Wright TA, Gray MR, Morris AI, et al. Cost effectiveness of detecting Barrett's cancer. *Gut* 1996; 39: 574-9.
37. Streitz JM, Ellis FH, Tilden RL, Erickson RV: Endoscopic surveillance of Barrett's esophagus: a cost-effectiveness comparison with screening mammography. *Am J Gastroenterol* 1996; 91: A71.
38. Spechler SJ, Goyal RK: Barrett's esophagus. *N Engl J Med* 1986; 315: 362-71.
39. Van Sandick JW, Van Lanschot JJB, Kuiken BW, Tytgat GNJ, Offerhaus GJA, Obertop H. Impact of endoscopic biopsy surveillance of Barrett's esophagus on pathological stage and clinical outcome of Barrett's carcinoma. *Gut* 1998; 43: 216-22.
40. Peters JH, Clark GW, Ireland AP, et al. Outcome of adenocarcinoma arising in Barrett's esophagus in endoscopically surveyed and non-surveyed patients. *J Thorac Cardiovasc Surg* 1994; 108: 813-21.
41. Cole P, Morrison AS: Basic issues in population screening for cancer. *J Natl Cancer Inst* 1980; 64: 1263-72.
42. Axon ATR, Boyle P, Riddell RH, et al. Summary of a working party on the surveillance of premalignant lesions. *Am J Gastroenterol* 1994; 89: S160-8.
43. Hutchison GB, Shapiro S. Lead time gained by diagnostic screening for breast cancer. *J Natl Cancer Inst* 1968; 41: 665-81.
44. Zelen M. Theory of early detection of breast cancer in the general population. In: Henson JC, Mattheiem WH, Rozencweig M, eds. *Breast cancer: trends in research and treatment*. New York: Raven Press, 1976: 287-300.
45. Pera M, Trastek VF, Carpenter HA, et al. Barrett's esophagus with high-grade dysplasia: an indication for esophagectomy? *Ann Thorac Surg* 1992; 54: 199-204.
46. Rice TW, Falk GW, Achkar E, Petras RE. Surgical management of high-grade dysplasia in Barrett's esophagus. *Am J Gastroenterol* 1993; 88: 1832-6.
47. Edwards MJ, Gable DR, Lentsch AB, Richardson JD. The rationale for esophagectomy as the optimal therapy for Barrett's esophagus with high-grade dysplasia. *Ann Surg* 1996; 223: 585-91.
48. Altorki NK, Sunagawa M, Little AG, Skinner DB. High-grade dysplasia in the columnar-lined esophagus. *Am J Surg* 1991; 161: 97-9.
49. Heitmiller RF, Redmond M, Hamilton SR. Barrett's esophagus with high-grade dysplasia. An indication for prophylactic esophagectomy. *Ann Surg* 1996; 224: 66-71.
50. Haggitt RC: Barrett's esophagus, dysplasia, and adenocarcinoma. *Hum Pathol* 1994; 25: 982-93.
51. Reid BJ, Weinstein WM, Lewin KJ, et al. Endoscopic biopsy can detect high-grade dysplasia or early adenocarcinoma in Barrett's esophagus without grossly recognizable neoplastic lesions. *Gastroenterology* 1988; 94: 81-90.

52. Levine DS, Haggitt RC, Blount PL, *et al*. An endoscopic biopsy protocol can differentiate high-grade dysplasia from early adenocarcinoma in Barrett's esophagus. *Gastroenterology* 1993; 105: 40-50.
53. Lee RG. Dysplasia in Barrett's esophagus. A clinicopathologic study of six patients. *Am J Surg Pathol* 1985; 9: 845-52.
54. Rothery GA, Patterson JE, Stoddard CJ, *et al*. Histological and histochemical changes in the columnar lined (Barrett's) esophagus. *Gut* 1986; 27: 1062-8.
55. Reid BJ, Haggitt RC, Rubin CE, *et al*. Correlation between flow cytometry and histology in detection of patients at risk for adenocarcinoma. *Gastroenterology* 1987; 93: 1-11.
56. Skinner DB, Walther BC, Riddell RH, *et al*. Barrett's esophagus, comparison of benign and malignant cases. *Ann Surg* 1983; 198: 554-65.
57. Menke-Pluymers MBE, Mulder AH, Hop WCJ, *et al*. Dysplasia and aneuploidy as markers of malignant degeneration in Barrett's esophagus. *Gut* 1994; 35: 1348-51.
58. DeMeester TR. Surgical treatment of dysplasia and adenocarcinoma. *Gastroenterol Clin North Am* 1997; 26: 669-84.
59. Hamilton SR, Smith RRL. The relationship between columnar epithelial dysplasia and invasive adenocarcinoma arising in Barrett's esophagus. *Am J Clin Pathol* 1987; 87: 301-12.
60. Schnell T, Sontag G, Chejfec G, *et al*. High-grade dysplasia in Barrett's esophagus: A report of the experience with 43 patients. *Gastroenterology* 1989; 96: 1746.
61. Schnell T, Sontag G, Chejfac G *et al*. High-grade dysplasia (HGD) is not an indication for surgery in patients with Barrett's esophagus. *Gastroenterology* 1996; 110: A590.
62. Levine DS, Haggitt RC, Blount PL, *et al*. An endoscopic biopsy protocol can differentiate high-grade dysplasia from early adenocarcinoma in Barrett's esophagus. *Gastroenterology* 1993; 105: 40-50.
63. Reid BJ, Blount PL, Rubin CE, *et al*. Flow-cytometric and histological progression to malignancy in Barrett's esophagus: Prospective endoscopic surveillance of a cohort. *Gastroenterology* 1992; 102: 1212-9.
64. Weston AP, Krmpotich PT, Cherian R, *et al*. Prospective long-term endoscopic and histological follow up of short segment Barrett's esophagus: Comparison with traditional long segment Barrett's esophagus. *Am J Gastroenterol* 1997; 92: 407-13.

Barrett's esophagus: new endoscopic strategies in case of dysplasia and early cancer

Christian Ell

Department of Internal Medicine II, Gastroenterology, Wiesbaden, Germany

Background

The incidence of adenocarcinoma of the esophagus has increased continuously during the last decades. Chronic acid reflux is strongly associated with adenocarcinoma of the esophagus and is the main cause of the development of specialised intestinal metaplasia in the esophagus (Barrett's esophagus). Barrett's esophagus is therefore considered a precancerous condition. Published data on malignant transformation in Barrett's esophagus show rates varying between 1 in 46 and 1 in 141 patients / years. More recent prospective data show that in Barrett's esophagus with histologically proven severe dysplasia adenocarcinoma subsequently develops in up to 34%.

The treatment of choice with curative intent has been esophagectomy. However, even at surgical centres that have sufficient experience and even, when patients are selected carefully, the mortality rates are in the range of 3% and 5% with Barrett's early carcinoma (EC) and high-grade dysplasia (HGD), respectively. There is a significant morbidity rate ranging from 18% to 48%. In view of these facts and because of the relatively large proportion of patients, who are unable to undergo surgery because of comorbidity or age, the question arises whether local endoscopic therapy might also be applicable in Barrett's EC and HGD, in analogy with early gastric cancer. Arguments in favour of intraluminal treatment by means of endoscopic techniques are as follows: morbidity and mortality should be essentially lower than in esophagectomy. With endoscopic techniques there is no major loss of quality of life. Furthermore, there are no risks for lymph node metastases in proven HGD and the risk for lymph nodes metastases is almost zero in patients with mucosal Barrett's cancer. Preliminary data negate, that in analogy to early gastric cancer, the lymph node metastases risk is very low, the same (probably 1-2%) in patients with Barrett's carcinoma from the submucosa level-I-type (SM 1 cancer). However, the lymph node metastases rate ranges between 10 and 20% in submucosal cancer of the 2nd and 3rd level (SM 2 and SM 3 cancer).

Staging procedures

In consequence, carefully designed staging procedures are necessary to find out preoperatively the patients with low risk for lymph node metastases, if local endoscopic treatment is scheduled. The staging procedures include - at least in our specialised centre - high-resolution video endoscopy with mapping biopsies, chromoendoscopy with methylen blue and biopsies of unstained or discolored lesions. A standard endosonography with 7.5 to 12 mHz is performed to detect lymph node enlargements in the mediastinum and the truncus coeliacus. In addition to mini-endosonography with through the scope probes with 20 mHz to investigate the infiltration depth of the tumor.

Abdominal ultrasound and spiral computed tomography of the thorax / mediastinum and the upper abdomen are oncological standards.

In some cases additional endoscopic mucosal resection is used for diagnostic purposes to get a clear information about the infiltration depth. Drug-induced or auto-fluorescence endoscopy are still experimental diagnostic methods.

The aims of the staging procedures are the exact mapping of the whole Barrett's segment; that means, detection of synchronous lesions, measurement of the diameter of the malignant lesion and furthermore description of the tumor surface as a polypoid (type I), flat (type II a, b, c) or ulcerated (type III). Concerning the infiltration depth we want to differentiate between mucosal type, submucosal type I, submucosal type II and III and, finally T2 tumors. Another important aim of the staging procedure is to get information about the tumor grading (G1 - G3).

In analogy to early gastric cancer we hope to define "low-risk Barrett's carcinoma" and HGD as follows: uni-locular lesions smaller than 2 cm, surface type I or II, infiltration type M or SM I, grading type G1 or G2 and lymph status negative.

Endoscopic treatment techniques

Three main endoscopic treatment techniques are available: endoscopic mucosal resection (EMR), photodynamic therapy (PDT) and thermoablation techniques as lasers and electrocoagulation. Details of the different treatment options can be obtained by the cited literature [1, 2].

Since all the treatment modalities have advantages and disadvantages, one should use a differentiated choice of the local treatment. Currently, we are using the EMR in about 60%, the PDT in about 30% and both, PDT in combination with EMR, in about 10%. Thermal methods should only be used for optimising the local endoscopic treatment and not as initial treatment.

Results

Currently there are only few published data on local endoscopic therapies of Barrett's EC and HGD. Besides some small casuistic series, there are only two groups with larger experiences: The Overholt group in USA reported on 100 patients with mainly high-grade dysplasia (> 70% HGD), treated exclusively by photodynamic therapy with hematoporphyrine derivates as photosensitizer. They achieved a local remission rate of about 80%, however, the rate of major complications was 34% and consisted in strictures of the esophagus which had to be treated by repeated dilation. In 1998 our own group reported about 32 patients with HGD and EC using amino levulinic acid. Due to the high concentration of the photosensitizer only in the mucosa and the short retention time in the body, severe side effects were never observed. However, the tumor destruction by this kind of PDT is limited to a maximum of 2 mm tissue depth. This circumstance was reflected by the results: we achieved a 100% complete remission rate in HGD but only 75% complete remission rate in EC. In the meantime we gathered experience with 70 patients altogether, treated by PDT (results not yet published). This year our group published a larger experience in endoscopic mucosal resection [3]: prospective investigation of EMR was conducted in 64 patients (61 patients with EC and 3 patients with HGD); 35 patients met the criteria for low risk. A total of 120 EMR was performed with only 1 major complication. A spurting bleeding could be managed endoscopically. Complete local remission was achieved significantly earlier in the low-risk group than in the high-risk group. A complete remission was achieved in 97% (34/35) of the patients in the low-risk group. In the high-risk group the complete remission rate was lower (59%). However, life table analyses showed that in this group a similar complete remission rate can also be expected after completion of all therapeutic steps.

Updated results of 114 out of 157 patients, who were treated locally in our center within the last 3 years (10/1996-9/1999) showed a complete remission rate of 98%. Only 2 patients were treatment failures and were treated by esophagectomy. The rate of major complications was 7%. During the follow-up of 18 months (mean) in 26 patients, metachronous lesions were detected and treated by endoluminal techniques again (the current results are not yet published).

Conclusions

Without any doubt radical surgical resection is still the treatment of choice for superficial Barrett's EC and HGD. Local endoscopic methods or intraluminal therapy are still experimental. However, the concept of local treatment is attractive because of the low morbidity, low mortality and the preservation of quality of life. The data currently available for intraluminal surgery show an excellent intermediate complete remission rate of more than 95%. However, long-term results have to be expected until esophagectomy will become the method of reserve.

References

1. Gossner L, Stolte M, Sroka R, Rick K, May A, Hahn EG, Ell C. Photodynamic ablation of high-grade dysplasia and early cancer in Barrett's esophagus by means of 5-aminolevulinic acid. *Gastroenterology* 1998; 114: 448-55.
2. Gossner L, May A, Stolte M, Seitz G, Hahn EG, Ell C. KTP laser destruction of dysplasia and early cancer in columnar-lined Barrett's esophagus. *Gastrointest Endosc* 1999; 49: 8-12.
3. Ell C, May A, Gossner L, Pech O, Günter E, Mayer G, Henrich R, Vieth M, Müller H, Seitz G, Stolte M. Endoscopic Mucosal Resection of Early Cancer and High-Grade Dysplasia in Barrett's Esophagus. *Gastroenterology* 2000; 118: 670-7.

II

Recent developments in gastro-intestinal oncology: colon cancer

Colon cancer screening

Morten H. Vatn[1], Geir Hoff[2], Espen Thiis-Evensen[2]

[1] Medical Department, Riks-Hospitalet University Hospital, Oslo, Norway ;
[2] Medical Department, Telemark Central Hospital, Skien, Norway

The reasons for proposing screening for colorectal cancer (CRC) are, first, that the disease is one of the major killers of Western societies [1, 2], second, that measures do exist, by which the mortality from the disease may be significantly reduced [3-5], third, that these measures may be accepted by the public [6], and, fourth, that they are acceptable in the light of cost benefit analysis [7]. Accepting that these requirements are generally met today by recent documentation, there still are several unresolved questions regarding how screening should be performed. Other problems are concerned with the relevance of extrapolating previous experience to other societies and populations. This overview will focus on the basic requirements for the planning of colorectal cancer screening, and on the discussion of the different screening methods available. Finally, the future aspects in science, with implementation of new technology for screening purposes, will be discussed.

How big is the problem?

On one side the size of the problem caused by the disease itself may be illustrated by the fact that the incidence of colorectal cancer has risen to more than 750 new cases per 1 million inhabitants in Western countries [1, 2]. Approximately 50% of these individuals will eventually die from their cancer after 5 years, in addition to quite a few after this period of time.

The fact that more than 90% of the new cases are sporadic does in fact limit our possibilities of primary prevention, as the frequency of inherited or familial cases presently are diagnosed only in 5-10% of cases. Under these circumstances, CRC detection and prevention is depending on clinical symptoms and signs in addition to secondary preventive measures (screening), since there is no documentation of any substantial effect of primary preventive measures.

Today, only fecal occult blood tests have shown a documented effect on mortality from CRC in large series. Nevertheless, these tests are hampered by high false positive and false negative rates. For this reason, and because invasive techniques are mandatory for verification and treatment, procedures that include visualization of the mucosa would also be more effective as screening tools, if not too costly or hazardous to the people.

Sigmoidoscopy provides an effective examination of the distal third of the large intestine [8], and would also cover the area mostly affected by CRC clinically. A larger proportion of the older patients with CRC located in the proximal part of the large intestine would eventually die from other causes. Nevertheless, at least 10-20% of the CRC lesions may be missed by ommitting the proximal parts of the colon at sigmoidoscopy, if there is no distal lesion. The lack of synchronicity between the presence of distal and proximal lesions, therefore, has formed the basis to suggest colonoscopy as the most sensitive test [9]. This again would increase the pressure on the demands for resources and highly skilled personel to keep up the standards of the procedures previously demonstrating the effect of screening in pilot studies.

Moreover, the inclusion of endoscopic procedures in screening of the average risk population needs some reflection. Not only does it imply demands on human and material resources, which would not replace, but, in fact, add to today's costs. One would also need to make sure that a population wide screening could be continued effectively, with a sufficient commitment by the public and health workers. A minimum of compliance by both sides is necessary to keep up the standards set at the introduction of the screening programme. We have to keep in mind that the alternative to organized screening procedures is "wild screening", where doctors are using different indications for examinations and follow-up of suspected cases. The costs of today's "wild screening" will have to be compared to the costs of organized screening as well.

The ideal model for a screening programme would be to demonstrate an effect of a prospective screening procedure in a pilot programme of the same population, which presently is being done in England, Norway and the US. These programmes should show an effect on the CRC mortality. One important requirement is that the programmes must be applicable to the routine practice of the community. It must be affordable with regard to extra resources. Each community must have the availability of personel, and between hospital networks for analysis of specimens. Standardization of histology and other screening analysis should be regarded. Also, the programme must be accepted by the population with regard to convenience and desire. Last but not least, the programme must include a plan to secure adequate handling of a follow-up created by the screening activity.

Evaluation of diagnostic tools

Because symptoms associated to the development of CRC are rather unspecific and signs often appearing too late for curable surgery, screening for early cancer or cancer precursor lesions is a tempting option. What screening tools are there?

Faecal occult blood tests (FOBT)

They represent the only modality that has been tested in adequate sized, controlled studies, to show a reduction in mortality of 15-18% for biennal screening, using unrehydrated Hemoccult-II slides in a randomized setting of the normal population [3, 4], and a 33% reduction using rehydrated slides in a population of volunteers [5]. The sensitivity of unrehydrated slides in a population screening has been estimated to be 54-62% [3], with a specificity of 98-99%. Unhydrated slides give 1-3% positive tests [3, 4] compared to 2-10% for rehydrated slides [5]. In the Minnesota trial, using rehydrated slides, this, combined with annual rather than biennial screening, exposed as much as 38% of screenees to colonoscopic follow-up [5] compared to 4% for the two other trials [3, 4]. Both false positive and false negative tests represent a problem when using guaiac-based FOBT. A more sensitive guaiac test, Hemoccult Sensa, reduces the false negative rates, but the positives went up. A combination, using an immunological test, HemSelect, to confirm a positive Hemoccult Sensa, has been reported to be beneficial [10].

In a study including non-malignant neoplasia, another immunochemical test, FlexSure OBT, with a performance very similar to HemSelect, was compared to Hemoccult Sensa and found to have a sensitivity for significant neoplasia of 35% compared to 50% (n.s.), and a specificity of 99% *versus* 95% in 1,410 individuals tested ($p < 0.05$) [11]. Similarly, the positive predictive value for Flexure OBT was 29% compared to 13% for Hemoccult Sensa. The advantage with FlexSure OBT is that it is easy and quick to perform, and to be read (after 5 minutes), with a distinct red line appearing when testing positive. It also tests positive at the presence of human blood only.

In general, since bleeding from colorectal lesions is intermittent, and since a benign neoplasia, such as the adenoma rarely bleeds, FOBT can in principle never be a test for adenoma detection. Therefore, screening with FOBT can never draw the full benefit of the proposed adenoma-carcinoma sequence of events to prevent CRC morbidity.

Endoscopic screening

It is based on the assumption that adenomas are the main precursors of CRC [12], and that their removal prevents progression to cancer. Although being practiced for decades, its efficacy still has to be evaluated in order to be accepted as an ideal screening tool in the average risk population. In general practice, the chances of detecting adenomas at endoscopy is generally independent of the indications for the procedure, and several decades after introduction of the procedure, no definite reduction of CRC has been observed in any of the Western countries.

Although the adenoma-carcinoma sequence theory [12] has never been directly proven, several studies have presented evidence substantiating the theory [9, 13-15]. In the US National Polyp Study [9], the incidence of CRC was 76 to 90% lower than expected after a complete colonoscopy with polypectomy in a cohort of 1,418 patients. A case control study [13] of 32,000 veterans showed that endoscopic procedures of the large intestine in conjunction with polyp removal reduced the risk of developing CRC by 50%. In another case-control study [14], rigid sigmoidoscopy reduced the mortality from cancer by 60%. In the most recent study of the effect of endoscopy with polypectomy among randomly chosen average risk individuals [15], the incidence of CRC was 1 among the 400 cases compared to 10 in the matched group of 400 controls, after more than 10 years of follow-up.

The basis for the understanding of the age-distribution of adenomas and its correlation to CRC was given by autopsy studies [16-18]. Based on one of these studies, by the use of a mathematical model, it was suggested that a screening strategy consisting of a baseline sigmoidoscopy at 60 years, with a follow-up of only 6% of the population, was estimated to prevent 50% of CRC's occurring after 60 years [19]. A range of alternative scenarios, giving rates of primary prevention of CRC from 40 to 70%, had costs which were comparable to those of breast-cancer screening, but was far superior considering effectivity.

Flexible sigmoidoscopy

Flexible sigmoidoscopy (FS) with polypectomy has been shown to be effective, long-term, for CRC prevention, only in one randomized study of the average risk population [15]. Several studies have included FS as an additional screening tool, in FOBT studies, to find that the pick-up rate to detect CRC and significant adenomas was significantly better for FS than for FOBT, in spite of a usually somewhat lower acceptance rate for FS than for FOBT [20-22]. As far as we know, attendance rates for FS in normal population screening has never been above 50%, except in the small Telemark Polyps study, with 81% attendance in 1983 [23], and in the ongoing, large scale Norwegian NORCCAP screening study in Oslo (57%) and Telemark (72%). In addition to high attendance rates, which are crucial, the performance of FS screening programmes depends on the age of the target population, the treshold for advancing to a baseline colonoscopy, and the availability of skilled personel to perform endoscopies.

With the same age group (55-64 years old), but a higher treshold for colonoscopies in the British "Once only flexible sigmoidoscopy-study" (adenomas > 10 mm at FS) than in the NORCCAP study (any adenoma), there is about 1 CRC diagnosed for each 300 individuals attending in both studies [23, 24]. This may just reflect that most CRCs are within the reach of FS, or it may indicate differences in the site distribution and incidence rates. Any community planning endoscopic screening should therefore have a thorough knowledge of these epidemiological aspects and carry out their pilot feasibility studies.

Colonoscopy

It has been suggested to be the most powerful screening tool against CRC. There is not only a site distribution shift towards the proximal colon with advancing age [18], this has also been observed as a time trend in Western societies independent of age. We also know that most adenomas regress and new ones will appear more proximally with increasing age. Thus, dependent on the local epidemiological situation and age of the target population, one may soon have to accept that the highest benefit may be achieved through colonoscopy screening, provided that attendance is sufficiently high, and that there is sufficient qualified personel available to perform examinations. It has been estimated that it requires 50% attendance rate for colonoscopy, 75% for FS and 90% for FOBT screening, respectively, to achieve 40% reduction in CRC mortality [7]. In the Telemark polyp study

[23], a 60% attendance rate was achieved when offering the full colonoscopy to a randomised sample of the normal population.

Regardless of choice of primary sigmoidoscopy or colonoscopy, one has to bear in mind that the sensitivity and specificity related to screening of the average risk population may vary to a great extent, as a consequence of its implementation in the given population.

It may be that the ideal screening procedure will consist of a differentiated offer of combined screening techniques as an alternative to total colonoscopy once or a few times during lifetime. Attempts are currently being made to evaluate cost-effectiveness and public acceptance of flexible endoscopy as a screening tool.

Cellular markers in faeces

Cellular markers in faeces, such as proteins or genetic markers, may be rational for screening purposes; however, there is a lack of documentation compared to the previously mentioned strategies. The results of research determining the molecular basis for colorectal cancer have lead to new suggestions of strategies that may be based on molecular markers. Examples of this are the detection of a series of defective DNA repair genes present in a high percentage of patients with hereditary CRC diseases [25, 26], and in as many as 15% of sporadic cases as well. A demonstration of the rational of screening in high-risk individuals was demonstrated in a comparison of mortality and incidence of CRC in asymptomatic at risk members of 22 families with HNPCC [27]. The results showed that screening at 3-year intervals by colonoscopy or barium enema, combined with flexible sigmoidoscopy, reduced the incidence of CRC in these high risk persons by 65%. Consequently, endoscopy and polypectomy seem to have the same protective effect against CRC in high risk as in average risk individuals.

The advantage of faecal markers in the screening of colorectal neoplasia is the avoidance of invasive and more costly examinations. Despite the recent documentation of a significantly reduced mortality by screening with Hemoccult, there is a need for tests with higher sensitivity and specificity. With modern technology, this is possible. Moreover, comparisons with blood testing is possible in large prospective trials, such as the ongoing Norwegian endoscopic screening study of average risk individuals, which has run from January 1999. In this study, 7,500 randomly chosen individuals, 55-63 years old, from each of two defined areas, are invited to endoscopy, eventually with polyppectomy, and testing of faecal samples, and compared with age and sex matched controls of the same areas.

Faecal markers for screening purposes may be classified as to their functional properties. They may represent different biochemical cathegories, such as carbohydrates, lipids, proteins, nucleic acids, or complex macromolecules, such as glycoproteins. The prerequisite must be that they can discriminate patients with colorectal neoplasia from those without. From a practical point of view, one may characterize markers on the basis of their way of acting in the gut lumen.

Characteristics of faecal markers

1. *Leakage from tumor* may be examplified by bleeding. Any bleeding may be considered as a marker, which apparently will lead to a low sensitivity and specificity. The sensitivity will further be reduced by the fact that bleeding generally occurs intermittently. Additionally, most adenomas will hardly ever bleed.

The specificity will be reduced because the blood will be derived from different sources, also from other areas of the bowel, in addition to the fact that the usual tests on faecal blood generally react to blood products in food. The FlexSure test, which is used in the NORCCAP-study, reacts only to human hemoglobin.

Even in CRC, bleeding occurs only in about 60% of cases. Calprotectin, a glycoprotein from white blood cells, has shown a higher rate of positive tests both in individuals with adenomas and carcinomas, compared to normal controls [28]. It resists degradation during transit through the bowel, is stable unfrozen during transport for up to a week [29], and may be stored frozen for at least one year (Axis Shield). Calprotectin must enter the lumen by other mechanisms than blood, since the correlation between these markers is low and since the "within patient variation" is much lower with calprotectin [30]. Even though Calprotectin is testing positive also in inflammatory conditions, this test may have a higher predictive value compared with FOBT. The use of Calprotectin as a screening tool may therefore, in spite of the tendency of false positive results, show an even higher reduction of deaths caused by CRC than FOBT, which so far is the only documented effective tool for screening of the average risk population. At the same time, comparison with secondary prophylaxis with endoscopy is important with regard to estimation of cost-effectiveness analysis. Testing for the detection of Calprotectin is performed with an Elisa technique, which is available and in practical use in several laboratories.

2. *Secretion or excretion from tumor* has the advantage compared to substances that leak (blood components) that they are directly related to cellular processes, which leads to continuous transport of markers from a tumor to the gut lumen. This leads to an increased specificity for the test. The most important substances of this category are substances from mucus [31]. Even if several of these substances must be regarded as interesting parameters, their significance has until now been greatly reduced by a substantial bacterial degradation in the gut lumen.

3. *Exfolliation of cells* from tumors represent potential markers of an optimal predictability for screening purposes. Nevertheless, these markers have been little examined. Close to a third of all cells from the mucosa are liberated daily in the gut lumen. Because adenomas have an increased turnover of cells compared to the normal mucosa, it has been estimated that adenomas with a diameter of 1 cm have a cell surface corresponding to about 1% of the colorectum, and that the surface of larger neoplasms is increasing exponentially to the increase in diameter [32, 33].

Cells from neoplasms and the normal mucosa may survive in the luminal surroundings and remain as intact cells during the entire transit time in the bowel [34, 35]. Thereby, intracellular markers may be protected against microorganisms in contrast to most non cell bound markers. It is also suspected that malignant cells have an advantage with regard to increased survival, due to a reduced tendency for apoptosis [36, 37]. In this way, cellular markers have a larger potential in relation to screening purposes for colorectal neoplasms.

It has for a long time been known that cytologic examinations of lavage fluid or oral bowel cleansing give a close to 100% sensitivity for CRC and a 95-100% specificity [38, 39]. By the use of fractionated sedimentation techniques, one has been able to obtain 10.6 cells per gram with more than 80% viability [34, 35]. The same studies also demonstrated that cells from all parts of the colorectum were present. The cytologic quality of colorectal cells have later been reproduced by others. In spite of this demonstration of a high reliability and discriminating value of cellular exfolliation, it must be stated that this method presently is impracticable for mass screening. Cytological examination of stools would represent a cumbersome method for mass screening due to a time consuming purification procedure and interpretation. The last developments in this field have focused on nuclear components, with examination of molecular genetic defects [40, 41]. The mutations that have been most intensively focused on, the APC-gene, k-ras and p53 mutations, do all have limitations with regard to sensitivity and specificity in relation to screening for CRC. Recent development of methods for quantitation of gene expression and mutation may, however, prove to increase the interest in these markers for CRC and large adenomas within the frames of mass screening. Possibly we may have to combine different sets of markers in the prevention of CRC. In addition to genetic markers, also cytoplasmatic enzymes [42, 43] and other proteins [39] have shown an over expression in CRC, dysplasia or large adenomas. It is possible that we, in addition to patterns of genetic changes, will have to look for combinations of RNA-associated changes and cytoplasmatic markers, which can tell us more about important characteristics of colorectal adenomas and cancer.

Complications to screening

To be justified, a screening procedure must have a low level of complications. In endoscopic examinations, one can expect complication rates such as haemorrhage and perforation, in the order of 0.1 to 2%, depending on whether any therapeutical interventions are performed [44, 45].

The possible negative psychological effect on the attendees has given rise to concern [46, 47]. Receiving a false positive result after a screening is invariably received with negative feelings. Individuals with a false positive mammography were shown to suffer from a high degree of anxiety that did not resolve immediately when new testing showed no signs of disease. In one study, 26% of women with an initially false positive mammogram had psychological disturbances affecting their mood, and 17% had their daily functioning affected 3 months after the mammography [48]. Increased anxiety for breast cancer was recorded up to 18 months after the examination that overruled the false positive result [49]. Even an invitation to a screening examination is known to inflict worry. It has been shown [50] that 15% of subjects invited to a faecal occult blood test experienced severe worries that could last for more than one week. A negative screening result is usually reassuring, but may have unwanted effects. It may reinforce an unhealthy lifestyle [51] and boost a pre-existing sense of invulnerability [52]. This "certificate of health effect" [51] may lead individuals who are screening negative for cancer to feel safe and continue smoking. Screening may also imply that good health can be maintained by regular "check-ups", leaving the individual behavior less important. A small adverse effect on quality of life, health promoting behavior, or the capacity to care for oneself, could have an impact on public health, outweighing the health gain achieved by screening. These aspects will have to be adressed in large-scale trials.

What have we learned from screening of CRC today?

In order to reach certain standards of population based screening, one has to combine our knowledge of the occurrence and development of CRC with the data from recent screening regimens performed in different countries. The main lessons to bring home as a basis for further achievements in the prevention of CRC are:
- CRC is age related, occurring mostly above 60 years,
- most CRC's occur in the average risk population in which high risk groups are poorly defined,
- only FOBT has been shown to reduce mortality from CRC in large trials,
- FOBT is hampered by false positive and false negative tests for CRC, and its performance is unsuitable for the detection of adenomas,
- pick-up rates for significant lesions at FS supersedes those of FOBT,
- primary prevention of CRC by endoscopy with polypectomy is indicated after the age of 55 in the average risk population,
- epidemiological trends may indicate a higher cost-effectiveness for colonoscopy than for FS screening in some populations,
- all cause mortality is not reduced in CRC screening studies.

Where do we go from here?

In order to improve the screening strategies, development of new modalities are needed:
- more specific genetic markers should be developed,
- the impact of combinations of markers should be evaluated in subsets of patients with increased adenoma or cancer risk,
- better characterization of risk groups should be performed, both for increased risk families and within today's average risk population,
- more differentiated follow-up programmes based on individual genetic and phenotypic profiles should be developed,
- the significance of flat adenomas should be validated further,
- increased need of endoscopic education should be considered a challenge for health care in the future,
- non invasive techniques, such as virtual colonoscopy, should be developed further,
- implementation of effective screening programmes should be performed on the basis of experience from ongoing large scale controlled screening programmes,
- the effect on all cause mortality and morbidity should be followed closely in all cohorts where systematic screening is implemented.

Conclusion

Screening for colorectal cancer and the precancerous adenoma is accepted as routine practice in Western societies today, especially on account of the documented decrease in mortality from CRC after FOBT screening. The cost-effectiveness is a major problem of this practice, due to great variation in sensitivity and specificity of the various tests. In spite of the general agreement stating that screening is a useful strategy, there is obviously room for improvement of effectiveness, partly due to limited knowledge of individual risk factors, partly to lack of resources for screening programmes and partly to problems with implementation in society.

To make future strategies more effective, one should be aiming at more selected strategies, more specific markers, better definition of subgroups and the lowest levels of somatic and psychological side effects. Valuable experience is expected from ongoing large-scale endoscopic screening programmes, which again will be awaiting competition from both sensitive and specific non-invasive techniques in the future.

References

1. Wingo PA, Tong T, Bolden S. Cancer statistics 1995. CA Cancer *J Clin* 1995; 155: 1741-8.
2. Cancer in Norway 1996. The Cancer Registry of Norway, Oslo 1999.
3. Hardcastle JD, Chamberlain JO, Robinson MH, Moss SM, Amar SS, Balfour TW. Randomized controlled trial of faecal-occult-blood-screening for colorectal cancer. *Lancet* 1996; 348: 1472-7.
4. Kronborg O, Fenger C, Olsen J, Jorgensen OD, Sondergaard O. Randomized study of screening for colorectal cancer with faecal- occult-blood test. *Lancet* 1996; 348: 1467-71.
5. Mandel JS, Church TR, Ederer F, Bond JH. Colorectal cancer. Mortality: Effectiveness of biennal screening for fecal occult blood. *J Natl Cancer Inst* 1999; 91: 434-7.
6. Thiis-Evensen E, Hoff GS, Sauar J, Majak BH, Vatn MH. The psychological effect of attending a screening program for colorectal cancer. *Scand J Gastroenterol* 1998; 34: 103.
7. Lieberman DA. Cost-effectiveness model for colorectal cancer Screening. *Gastroenterology* 1995; 109: 1781-90.
8. Hoff GS, Vatn MH. Epidemiology of polyps in the rectum and sigmoid colon. Endoscopic evaluation of size and localization of polyps. *Scand J Gastroenterol* 1985; 20: 356-60.
9. Winawer S, Zauber AG, Ho MN, O'Brien MJ, Gottlieb L, Stern-Berg SS, Waye JD, Schapiro M, Bond JH, Panish JF, Ackroyd F, Shike M, Kurz RC, Hornsby-Lewis L, Gerdes H, Stewart ET and the National Polyp Study workgroup. Prevention of colorectal cancer by colonoscopic polypectomy. *N Engl J Med* 1993; 329: 1977-8.
10. Allison JE. Review article: faecal occult blood testing for colorectal cancer. *Aliment Pharmacol Ther* 1998; 12: 1-10.
11. Rozen P. Colorectal cancer screening in Israel. *Gastrointest Endosc* 1998; 47: 97-100.
12. Muto T, Bussey HJ, Morson BC. The evolution of cancer of the colon and rectum. *Cancer* 1975; 36: 2251-70.
13. Müller AD, Sonnenberg A. Prevention of colorectal cancer by flexible endoscopy and polypectomy. A case control study of 32,702 veterans. *Ann Intern Med* 1995; 42: 109-13.
14. Selby JV, Friedman GD, Quesenberry PC Jr, Weiss NS. A case Control study of screening sigmoidoscopy and mortality from colorectal cancer. *N Engl J Med* 1992; 326: 653-7.

15. Thiis-Evensen E, Hoff GS, Sauar J, Langmark F, Majak BM, Vatn MH. Population based surveillance by colonoscopy: Effect on the incidence of colorectal cancer. *Scand J Gastroenterol* 1999; 34: 414-20.
16. Arminski TC, Mc Lean DW. Incidence of adenomatous polyps of the colon and rectum based on 1,000 autopsy examinations. *Dis Colon Rectum* 1964; 7: 249-61.
17. Eide JT, Stalsberg H. Polyps of the large intestine in Northern Norway. *Cancer* 1978; 4 (2): 2839-48.
18. Vatn MH, Stalsberg H. The prevalens of polyps of the large intestine in Oslo. An autopsy study. *Cancer* 1982; 49: 819-25.
19. Geul KW, Bosman FT, van Blankenstein M, Grobbee DE, Wilson JHP. Prevention of colorectal cancer: costs and effectiveness of sigmoidoscopy. *Scand J Gastroenterol* 1997; 32 (Suppl. 223): 79-87.
20. Verne J, Aubrey R, Love SB, Talbot IC, Northover JMA. Population based randomised study of uptake and yield of screening by flexible sigmoidoscopy compared with screening by faecal occult blood testing. *Br Med J* 1998; 3 (17): 182-5.
21. Rasmussen M, Kronborg O, Fenger C, Jørgensen OD. Possible advantages and drawbacks of adding flexible sigmoidoscopy to Hemoccult-II in screening for colorectal cancer. *Scand J Gastroenterol* 1999; 34: 73-8.
22. Brevinge H, Lindholm E, Buntzen S, Kewenter J. Screening for colorectal neoplasia with faecal occult blood testing compares with flexible sigmoidoscopy directly in a 55-56 years old population. *Int J Colorectal Dis* 1997; 12: 291-5.
23. Hoff GS, Vatn MH, Gjone E, Larsen S, Sauar J. Epidemiology of Polyps in the rectum and sigmoid colon. *Scand J Gastroenterol* 1985; 20: 351-5.
24. Atkin WS, Cuzick J, Northover JM, Whynes DK. Prevention of colorectal cancer by once-only sigmoidoscopy. *Lancet* 1993; 341: 736-40.
25. Fishel R, Lescoe MK, Rao MR, Copeland NG, Jenkins NA, Garber J. The human mutator gene homolog MSH2 and its association with hereditary non-polyposis colon cancer. *Cell* 1993; 75: 1027-38.
26. Bronner CE, Baker SM, Morrison PT, Warren G, Smith LG, Lescoe MK. Mutation in the DNA mismatch repair gene homologue hMLH1 in association with heriditary non-polyposis colon cancer. *Nature* 1994; 368: 258-61.
27. Järvinen HJ, Mecklin JP, Sistonen P. Screening reduces colorectal cancer rate in families with hereditary nonpolyposis colorectal cancer. *Gastroenterology* 1995; 108: 1405-11.
28. Kristinsson J, Røseth A, Fagerhol M, Aadland E, Schjønsby H, Børmer OP, Nygaard K. Fecal calprotectin concentration in patients with colorectal carcinoma. *Dis Colon Rectum* 1998; 41: 316-21.
29. Roseth A, Fagerhol M, Aadland E, Schjonsby H. Assessment of the neutrophil dominating protein calprotectin in feces: a methodologic study. *Scand J Gastroenterol* 1992; 27: 793-8.
30. Gilbert JA, Ahlquist D, Mahony DW, Zinsmeister AR, Rubin J, Ellefson RD. Fecal marker variability in colorectal cancer: calprotectin versus hemoglobin. *Scand J Gastroenterol* 1996; 31: 1001-6.
31. Itzkowitz SH, Bloom EJ, Kokal WA, Modin G, Hakomori S, Kim YS. Sialosyl T. A novel mucin antigen associated with poor prognosis in colorectal cancer patients. *Cancer* 1990; 66: 1960-6.
32. Quirke P, Dixon MF, Clayden AD. Aneuploidy and cell proliferation in rectal adenocarcinoma. *J Pathol* 1987; 151: 285-91.
33. Shorter RG, Moertel CG, Titus JL, Rietmeier RJ. Cell kinetics in the jejunum and rectum of man. *Am J Dig Dis* 1964; 9: 760-3.
34. Lyengar V, Albaugh GP, Lohani A, Nair PP. Human stools as a source of viable colonic epithelial cells. *FASEB* 1991; 5: 2856-9.
35. Albaugh GP, Lyngear V, Lohani A. Isolation of exfoliated colonic epithelial cells, a novel noninvasive approach to the study of human cellular markers. *Int J Cancer* 1992; 52: 347-50.
36. Iwanaga T, Han H, Adachi K, Fujita T. A novel mechanism for disposing of effete epithelial in the small intestine. *Gastroenterology* 1993; 105: 1089-97.
37. Bedi A, Pasricha PJ, Akthar T. Inhibition of apoptosis during the development of colorectal cancer. *Cancer res* 1995; 55: 1811-6.

38. Gordon IL, Rypsin EB, Wuerker RB, Janowatz JJ. Cytologic detection of colorectal cancer after administration of oral lavage solution. *Cancer* 1991; 68: 106-10.
39. Darmon E, Tobi M, Rozen P. Newer tests in the colonic effluent for identifying persons with colorectal neoplasia. In: Rozen P, Reich CB, Winawer SJ, eds. *Large bowel cancer: policy, prevention, research, and treatment.* Basel-Karger, 1991: 236-47.
40. Feraron ER, Vogelstein B. A genetic model for colorectal tumorigenesis. *Cell* 1990; 61: 759-67.
41. Scott N, Quirke P. Molecular biology of colorectal neoplasia. *Gut* 1993; 34: 289-92.
42. Vatn MH, Jellum E, Elgjo K, Bergan A. Enzyme activity and protein patterns as premalignant markers in mucosal biopsies of the large intestine. *Scand J Gastroenterol* 1985; (Suppl. 20) 107: 1-7.
43. Jellum E, Thorsrud AK, Vatn MH, Grimstad I, Brennhovd I, Tveit KM, Pihl A. Detection of cancer related proteins by two-dimensional electrophoresis. *Ann NY Acad Sci* 1984; 428: 173-85.
44. Habr-Gama A, Waye JD. Complications and hazards of gastrointestinal endoscopy. *World J Surg* 1989; 13: 193-201.
45. Winawer SJ, Fletcher RH, Miller R. Colorectal cancer screening: clinical guidelines and rationale. *Gastroenterology* 1997; 112: 594-602.
46. Stewart-Brown S, Farmer A. Screening could seriously damage your health. Editorial. *Br Med J* 1997; 314: 533-4.
47. Marteau TM. Psychological costs of screening. Editorial. *Br Med J* 1989; 299: 527.
48. Lerman C, Trock B, Rimer BK. Psychological and behavioural implications of abnormal mammograms. *Ann Intern Med* 1991; 114: 657-61.
49. Gram IT, Lund E, Slenker SE. Quality of life following a false positive mammogram. *Br J Cancer* 1990; 62: 1018-22.
50. Lindholm E, Berglund B, Haglin E. Worry associated with screening for colorectal carcinomas. *Scand J Gastroenterol* 1997; 32: 238-45.
51. Tymstra T, Bieleman B. The psychological impact of mass screening for cardiovascular risk factors. *Fam Pract* 1987; 4: 287-90.
52. Weinstein ND. Why it won't happen to me: perceptions of risk factors and susceptibility. *Health Psychol* 1984; 3: 431-57.

Primary prophylaxis of colon cancer: what is established?

Meinhard Classen, Eckart Frimberger

Department of Internal Medicine II, Technical University, Munich, Germany

About 5-6% of the US population will develop colorectal cancer. There is epidemiological evidence that both environmental (diet, physical activity) and genetic (family history, germline mutations and polymorphisms) factors are related to cancer risk [1]. Because colorectal cancers usually arise from adenomatous polyps it is thought that preventing the growth of adenomas will prevent colorectal cancer [2, 3]. Evidence has accumulated that the growth of colorectal adenomas and carcinomas may be prevented by nutrition and by chemopreventive agents. The term "chemoprevention" was introduced to define "the prevention of cancer by the use of pharmacological agents that inhibit or reverse the process of carcinogenesis [4].

Nutrition and cancer prevention

Observational studies

Dietary recommendations for the reduction of cancer risk are based on data from observational studies of the relationship between diet and cancer incidence [5, 6]. Findings from observational epidemiologic studies suggest that diets high in fruit and vegetables are associated with lower risk for cancer at many sites, especially in the gastrointestinal tract [5, 6]. In 1981, Doll and Peto estimated that about 35% of all cancers in the US might be related to dietary factors [7]. Similar estimates were made by others [6, 8].

Randomised controlled trials

Relationships between nutrients and cancer risk have now been studied in a number of completed randomised controlled trials.

A Medline search of the National Library of Medicine's PubMed system (www.pubmed.gov) was conducted to examine published studies of nutrition and cancer that used a randomized controlled design. Included in this review are all papers or abstracts published in English that reported study designs featuring a random assignment of foods or nutrients to at least 200 people (to eliminate under-powered studies) and that examined cancer or colorectal adenomatous polyps as the study endpoint. Not included were studies of non-nutritive synthetic compounds or of various intermediate biomarkers of neoplasia risk (*e.g.* proliferation, dysplasia, or cytologic atypia) [9]. The findings are summarized in *table I*.

Table I. Randomised controlled trials of various nutrients and the incidence of cancers and adenomatous polyps. Adapted from [9].

Study or investigator	Nutrients tested, daily dose	Years on study	Relative risk (agent *vs* placebo)
Colorectal cancer			
NPSC* [11]	Selenium 200 mcg	5	0.42
ATBC* [10]	Beta carotene 20 mg	6	1.05
ATBC* [10]	Vitamin E 50 IU	6	0.83
Colorectal adenomas			
McKeown-Eyssen [12]	Cereal fiber 20 g	2	1.2
MacLennan [13]	Cereal fiber 25 g	4	1.2
MacLennan [13]	Beta carotene 20 mg	4	1.5
Greenberg [14]	Beta carotene 25 mg	4	1.01
Greenberg [14]	Vitamin E 400 IU + Vitamin C 1 gm	4	1.08
Baron [15]	Calcium 1.2 gm	4	0.83
Bonelli [16]	Selenium 200 mcg	4	0.56

Colorectal cancer, adenomas

Two trials of nutritional supplementation have reported colorectal cancer endpoints, but neither included colorectal cancer as one of the *a priori* primary endpoints. Neither beta carotene nor vitamin E appeared to affect colorectal cancer risk in the Alpha Tocopherol Beta Carotene study [10]. In the Nutritional Prevention of Skin Cancer study, colorectal cancer was seen less frequently in the intervention group [11].

Several studies have used a clinical model to examine the impact of nutritional supplements on the formation of adenomatous polyps in the colon and rectum. Patients undergoing a polypectomy with a cleansing colonoscopy are randomized to intervention *versus* placebo groups. The efficacy of the nutritional supplement is estimated by the relative rates of new adenomas detected in the two groups at the time of their follow-up colonoscopy three years later.

New polyp growth was not affected by wheat bran fiber supplements in two studies [12, 13] or in studies testing anti-oxidants, singly [13] or in combination [14]. In one trial, calcium supplementation was associated with a 17% reduction in the rate of new polyp formation [15]. This effect is thought to be related to the binding of calcium to bile acids, making them less likely to stimulate growth in the colonic mucosa. To test the observation that selenium appeared to reduce the incidence of colorectal cancer, the polyp prevention trial design was used; a 44% reduction in the incidence of new polyp growth was found in the selenium arm of the study [16].

In a recent randomized trial [17] the effect of dietary supplementation with wheat-bran fiber on the rate of recurrence of colorectal adenomas was investigated; 1,303 subjects who were 40 to 80 years of age completed the study. They had one or more colorectal adenomas removed within three months before recruitment to a supervised program of dietary supplementation with either high amounts (13.5 g per day) or low amounts (2 g per day) of wheat-bran fiber. The median times from randomization to the last follow-up colonoscopy were 34 and 36 months. Neither in the low-fiber group nor in the high-fiber group a protective effect against recurrent colorectal adenomas was found.

In another recent randomized trial [18] the effect of a low-fat, high-fiber diet on the recurrence of colorectal adenomas was investigated; 1,905 subjects, mean age 61 years, who had one or more colorectal adenomas removed within six months before randomization, completed the study. For the subjects in the intervention group, the dietary goals were to provide 20% of total calories from fat, 18 g of dietary fiber per 1,000 kcal, and 3.5 servings of fruits and vegetables per 1,000 kcal. The intervention program included nutritional information and behavior-modification techniques. Subjects in the control group were provided with general dietary guidelines but not given additional nutritional or behavioral information. The subjects were followed for approximately four years after randomization. The study provided no evidence that a diet low in fat and high in fiber, fruit, and vegetables reduces the risk of recurrent colorectal adenomas.

Chemoprevention

Animal studies, human epidemiological studies and clinical studies suggest that nonsteroidal antiinflammatory drugs, NSAID, may be potent agents for the prevention of colorectal cancer.

NSAID inhibit the prostaglandin synthesis by direct inhibition of cyclooxygenase (COX) enzymes. NSAID inhibit the cyclooxygenase enzymes which regulate the conversion of arachidonic acid to prostaglandins. At least two isoforms of COX exist. COX-1 is present in the normal gastrointestinal mucosa. Inhibition of COX-1 in the gastroduodenal mucosa by NSAID may cause NSAID-induced ulcers. COX-2 is not detectable in the normal gastrointestinal mucosa but its expression can be induced by growth factors. Upregulation of COX-2 expression has been found in adenomas and carcinomas [19]. It was shown in rats that a selective COX-2 inhibitor had chemopreventive activity in the aberrant crypt focus induced with azoxymethane [20]. The lack of COX-2 expression in the normal colonic mucosa and its overexpression in colonic neoplasia explains the selective action of COX-2 inhibitors on neoplastic colonic mucosa without the risk of gastroduodenal ulcers [1]. Several recently developed selective COX-2 inhibitors, celecoxib, nimesulide and others, are under evaluation as chemopreventive agents [21, 22]. The chemopreventive action of NSAID-type drugs is probably not exclusively mediated by their action on COX-2.

Animal studies

Animal studies have shown that NSAID, *e.g.* indomethacin and sulindac prevent carcinogen-induced colonic carcinogenesis [23-27]. They may have a preventive effect even when given 14 weeks after the carcinogen [25]. Part of the preventive effect occurs early in carcinogenesis as the formation and/or growth of aberrant crypt foci which seems to be the earliest histological lesion in the neoplastic process is inhibited [26]. NSAIDs also inhibit adenoma formation in the Min-mouse, the animal model of familial adenomatous polyposis (FAP) [27].

Patients with familial adenomatous polyposis

The effect of sulindac on colonic adenomas in FAP patients was shown in an open-labelled study [28, 29]. In subsequent controlled trials, the dramatic regression of existing adenomas and prevention of new adenomas in FAP were confirmed [30, 31].

Descriptive epidemiology

The relationship between regular NSAID use and risk of colon cancer has been studied in numerous cohort and case control studies. The results of 14 trials are shown in *figure 1*.

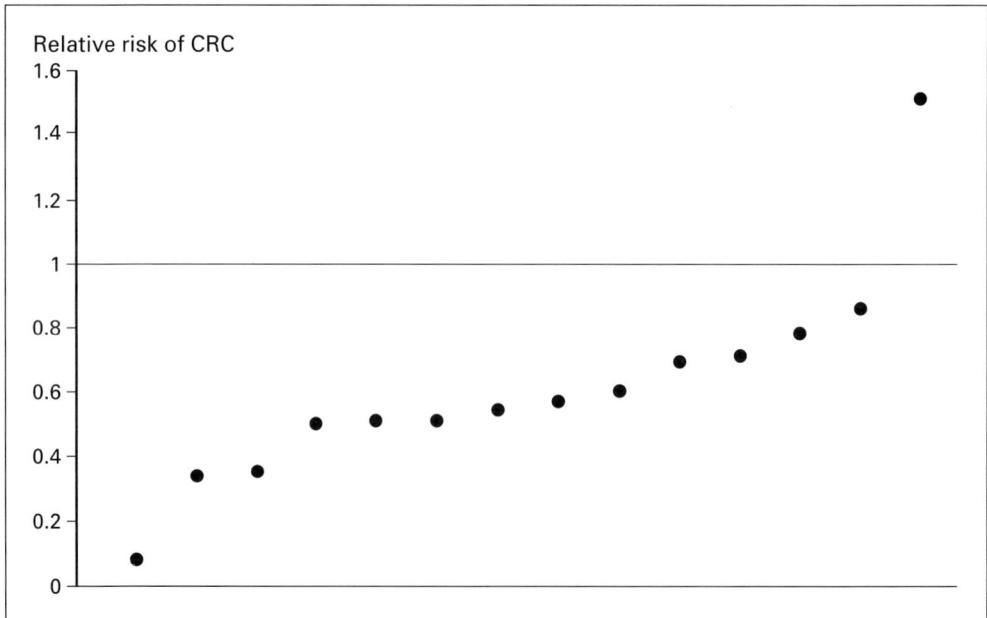

Figure 1. Relative risk of CRC or colonic adenomas in regular NSAID users *versus* non-users from 14 case control and cohort studies. From [1], data drawn from studies cited in [24, 25, 32, 33, 39, 40].

In the majority of the trials a protective relationship between regular NSAID use and either colon death rate or adenoma recurrence rate was found. The average reduction in relative risk is about 0.5 for regular NSAID users *vs* non-users and the protective effect was generally seen in all age groups included, and in both men and women [1]. Most studies had insufficient data to clarify the relationship between dose and duration of NSAID use and risk of colorectal cancer. The American Cancer Society Study [32] and the Nurses Health Study [33] suggested that a relatively low dose, three or four tablets per week, was preventive. In the Nurses Health Study also, a strong relationship between the duration of ASA use and CRC risk was found. No risk reduction was seen until more than 10 years of ASA use and the relationship was not significant until 20 years of use *figure 2*.

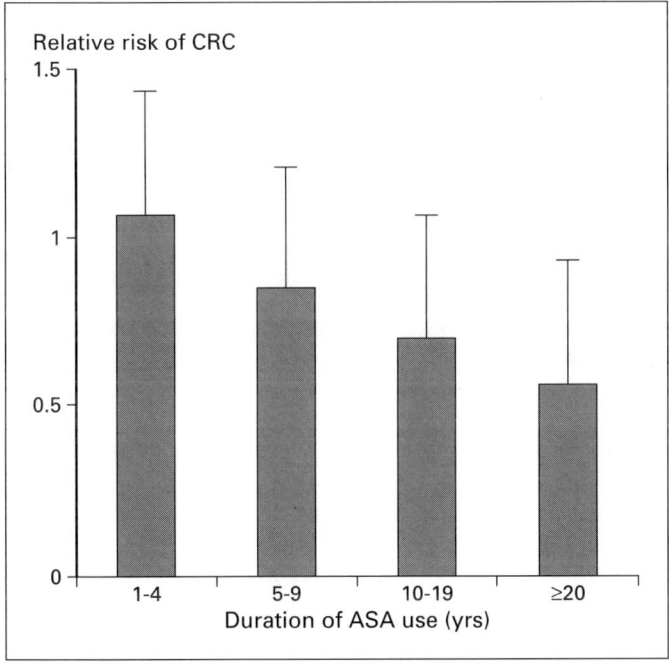

Figure 2. Relative risk of colorectal cancer in regular aspirin users as a function of the duration of aspirin use. From [33].

Intervention trials

In a large intervention trial, the Physicians Health Study (PHS), one aspirin tablet (325 mg) every other day during 5 years was included as one of the intervention arms [24]. There was no significant decrease in the incidence of either colonic adenomas or carcinomas in the aspirin-group. In two small NSAID polyp regression studies [34, 35], eligible subjects with small polyps in the left colon were enrolled. The polyps were tattooed and left in place. In one of the studies in which subjects were treated with an NSAID or placebo, little evidence was found for polyp regression. In the other trial comparing placebo to sulindac at either 150 or 300 mg *per* day, a significant reduction in the number of subjects who had adenoma growth during 12 months of treatment was reported.

Conclusion

Findings from observational epidemiologic studies support the notion that diets high in fruit and vegetables are associated with lower risk for cancer at many sites, especially in the gastrointestinal tract. However, estimates from these studies are considered imprecise because observational nutritional research is plagued by uncertainties about dietary assessment methodology [9].

Randomized controlled trials are considered as much more definitive than are observational studies with respect to causality. They eliminate the problems of dietary recall and control the effects of both known and unknown confounding factors. However, many randomized controlled trials of nutrition and cancer that have been completed to date have largely followed the investigational paradigm of pharmacology--testing single nutrients in super-nutritional doses [9].

It is difficult to test whole food or whole-diet interventions in randomized controlled trial designs, and it cannot be done in a blinded way. Such trials usually study individuals at high risk of neoplasia for short periods of time. As if we were searching for a new therapeutic compound, we have expected high doses of a single nutrient to reproduce the beneficial effects of the complex nutrient mixtures found in whole food. Perhaps this basic assumption is wrong. The first generation of randomized controlled trials of antioxidant nutrients has not shown any substantial benefit thus far with most of the nutritional supplements tested. There are only a few exceptions: a modest reduction of colorectal adenomatous polyp growth with calcium supplementation [15], and effects of selenium on colorectal cancers [11, 36].

The possible role of nutrients as protective factors in the later phases of the transition of adenomas to cancer cannot be easily studied in the polyp trial designs, as they focus only on the first one to three years of new polyp growth following the removal of a metachronous polyp. Problematic is our inability to study later phases of colorectal cancer development when large adenomatous polyps devolve to cancer. Trials in which adenomas are left in place are ethically difficult, although one such small trial was recently reported [37].

Disappointing results from randomized controlled trials including the two most recent ones [17, 18] have shown us that the use of some of the diets and nutritional supplements has no short term benefits with respect to preventing adenomas [3]. In the context of the long course of the evolution of colorectal carcinoma, the three- or four-year period assessed by clinical studies is very brief [3, 38]. It is therefore appropriate to question the relevance of these trials for the prevention of colorectal cancer. With regard to questions about diet and colorectal cancer, though, definitive answers still seem to be beyond the reach of both observational epidemiologic studies and randomized, controlled trials [3].

Observational studies around the world continue to find that the risk of colorectal cancer is lower among populations with high intakes of fruit and vegetables and that the risk changes on adoption of a different diet, but we still do not understand why [3, 5, 6]. It is unclear whether a single aspect of the diet - a particular vitamin, phytochemical, or dietary practice such as the method of cooking meats -accounts for this relation [3].

There remains compelling evidence that eating five or more servings of fruit and vegetables per day can substantially reduce the risk of some of the most commonly occurring cancers in the US. The combined effects of nutrients as contained in the mixtures commonly known as whole food seem to be more effective in reducing cancer risk than are nutrients contained in supplements [5, 6]. This simple conclusion can be a sound basis for broad nutritional advice to the population, as well as for clinical counselling of individual patients.

In the future, randomized controlled trials will need to incorporate lessons learned in early trials. It would seem wise to test the effects of nutritional supplements given in broader combinations, and in more modest doses, thereby simulating the micronutrient combinations in the matrix of whole food. Trials should also be designed to be long-term, testing nutrients over many years among people at average risk. Individuals who are at high risk because of factors such as specific carcinogen exposure, familial history, or the existence of a premalignant lesion, may be generally less susceptible to nutrient effects than are those at average risk. Consequently, it may be unwise to study only those at high risk.

Descriptive epidemiology indicates a strong association between long-term, regular ASA use and a decreased rate of neoplasia. However, such studies can only establish an association, they cannot prove that the association is causal [1].

In an intervention trial, the Physicians Health Study, the incidence of either colonic adenomas or carcinomas was not influenced by aspirin. The aspirin intervention may have been too short (5 years) or the dose may have been too low (325 mg) to reduce incidence of colonic neoplasia.

The risk profile of standard NSAID remains a problem. The risk of gastrointestinal toxicity is directly related to the age of the population treated [1]. This has led to great interest in the chemopreventive potential of selective COX-2 inhibitors and of NSAID metabolits not inhibiting either COX-1 or COX -2 because gastrointestinal ulceration is thought to be related to COX-1.

In summary, current evidence suggests that NSAIDs inhibit colonic carcinogenesis. Additional intervention trials are necessary to determine if the NSAID effect is not only limited to FAP-subjects but also to subjects with sporadic adenomas and to determine the most effective and safe dose and the duration of use necessary for prevention. At present no confident recommendation can be made for the widespread use of NSAIDs to prevent colorectal cancer [1].

References

1. Ahnen DJ. Colon cancer prevention by non-steroidal antiinflammatory drugs. What is evidence? What is the mechanism of action? In: W Schmiegel, J Schölmerich, eds. *Colorectal cancer*. Dordrecht; Boston, London: Kluwer Academic Publishers, 1998.
2. Winawer SJ, Fletcher RH, Miller L, *et al.* Colorectal cancer screening: clinical guidelines and rationale. *Gastroenterology* 1997; 112: 594-642.

3. Byers T. Diet, colorectal adenomas, and colorectal cancer. *N Engl J Med* 2000; 342: 1206-7 (editorial).
4. Sporn MB, Newton DL. Chemoprevention of cancer with retinoids. *Fed Procs* 1979; 38: 2528-34.
5. The American Cancer Society 1996 Advisory Committee on Diet, Nutrition, and Cancer Prevention. Guidelines on diet, nutrition, and cancer prevention: Reducing the risk of cancer with healthy food choices and physical activity. *CA Cancer J Clin* 1996; 46: 325-41.
6. World Cancer Research Fund in association with American Institute for Cancer Research: Food, Nutrition, and the Prevention of Cancer: A Global Perspective. Washington, DC: American Institute for Cancer Research, 1997.
7. Doll R, Peto R. The causes of cancer. Quantitative estimates of avoidable risks of cancer in the United States today. *J Natl Cancer Inst* 1981; 66: 1191-308.
8. Miller A, Berrino F, Hill M, et al. Diet in the aetiology of cancer: A review. *Eur J Cancer* 1994; 30A: 207-20.
9. Byers T. What Can Randomized Controlled Trials Tell Us About Nutrition and Cancer Prevention? *CA Cancer J Clin* 1999; 49: 353-61.
10. The Alpha-Tocopherol, Beta-Carotene Prevention Study Group. The effect of vitamin E and beta-carotene on the incidence of lung cancer and other cancers in male smokers. *N Engl J Med* 1994; 330: 1029-35.
11. Clark LC, Combs GF Jr, Turnbull BW, et al. Effects of selenium supplementation for cancer prevention in patients with carcinoma of the skin: A randomized controlled trial: Nutritional Prevention of Cancer Study Group. *JAMA* 1996; 276: 1957-63.
12. McKeown-Eyssen GE, Bright-See E, Bruce WR, et al. A randomized trial of a low fat high fiber diet in the recurrence of colorectal polyps. *J Clin Epidemiol* 1994; 47: 525-36.
13. MacLennan R, Macrae F, Bain C, et al. Randomized trial of intake of fat, fiber, and beta carotene to prevent colorectal adenomas: The Australian Polyp Prevention Project. *J Natl Cancer Inst* 1995; 87; 1760-6.
14. Greenberg ER, Baron JA, Tosteson TD, et al. A clinical trial of antioxidant vitamins to prevent colorectal adenoma: Polyp Prevention Study Group. *N Engl J Med* 1994; 331: 141-7.
15. Baron J, Beach M, Mandel J, et al. Calcium supplements for the prevention of colorectal adenoma. *N Engl J Med* 1999; 340: 101-7.
16. Bonelli L, Conio M, Massa P, et al. Chemoprevention with antioxidants of metachronous adenomas of the large bowel. *Cancer Prevention and Control* 1998; 100: A351.
17. Alberts DS, Martinez ME, Roe DJ, et al. Lack of effect of a high-fiber cereal supplement on the recurrence of colorectal adenomas. *N Engl J Med* 2000; 342: 1156-62.
18. Schatzkin A, Lanza E, Corle D, et al. Lack of effect of a low fat, high- fiber diet on the recurrence of colorectal adenomas. *N Engl J Med* 2000; 342: 1149-55.
19. Eberhart CE, Coffey RJ, Radhika A, et al. Up-regulation of cyclooxygenase 2 gene expression in human colorectal adenomas and adenocarcinomas. *Gastroenterology* 1994; 107: 1183-8.
20. Reddy BS, Rao CV, Seibert K. Evaluation of cyclooxygenase-2 inhibitor for potential chemopreventive properties in colon carcinogenesis. *Cancer Res* 1996; 56: 4566-71.
21. Donelly MT, Hawkey CJ. Review article: COX-II inhibitors - a new generation of safer NSAIDS? *Aliment Pharmacol Ther* 1997; 11: 227-36.
22. Decensi A, Costa A. Recent advances in cancer chemoprevention, with emphasis on breast and colorectal cancer. *Eur J Cancer* 2000; 36: 694-709.
23. Marnett LJ. Aspirin and related non-steroidal anti-inflammatory drugs as chemopreventive agents against colon cancer. *Prev Med* 1995; 24: 103-6.
24. Gann PH, Manson JE, Glynn RJ, Hennekens CH. Low-dose aspirin and incidence of colorectal tumors in a randomized trial (see comment). *J Natl Cancer Inst* 1993; 85: 1220-4.

25. Reddy BS, Maruyama H, Kellof G. Dose-related inhibition of colon carcinogenesis by dietary piroxicam, a nonsteroidal antiinflammatory drug, during different stages of rat colon tumor development. *Cancer Res* 1987; 47: 5340-6.
26. Wargovic MJ, Chen CD, Harris C, et al. Inhibition of aberrant crypt growth by non-steroidal anti-inflammatory agents and differentiation agents in the rat colon. *Int J Cancer* 1995; 60: 515-9.
27. Beazer-Barclay Y, Levy DB, Moser AR, et al. Sulindac supresses tumorigenesis in the Min mouse. *Carcinogenesis* 1996; 17: 1757-60.
28. Waddell WR, Loughry RW. Sulindac for polyposis of the colon. *J Surg Oncol* 1983; 24: 83-7.
29. Waddell WR, Ganser GF, Cerise EJ, Loughry RW. Sulindac for polyposis of the colon. *Am J Surg* 1989; 157: 175-9.
30. Labayle D, Fisher D, Vielh P, et al. Sulindac causes regression of rectal polyps in familial adenomatous polyposis. *Gastroenterology* 1991; 101: 635-9.
31. Giardiello FM, Hamilton SR, Krush AJ. Treatment of colonic and rectal adenomas with sulindac in familial adenomatous polyposis. *N Engl J Med* 1993; 328: 1313-6.
32. Thun MJ, Namboodiri MH, Heath CW. Aspirin use and reduced risk of fatal colon cancer. *N Engl J Med* 1991; 325: 1593-6.
33. Giovanucci E, Egan KM, Hunter DJ, et al. Aspirin and the risk of colorectal cancer in women. *N Engl J Med* 1995: 333: 609-14.
34. Hixson LJ, Earnest DL, Fennerty MB, Sampliner RE. NSAID effect on sporadic colon polyps. *Am J Gastroenterol* 1993; 88: 1652-6.
35. Disario JA, Alberts ES, Tietze CC, et al. Sulindac induces regression and prevents progression of sporadic colorectal adenomas. *Gastroenterology* 1977; 112: A555 (abstract).
36. Clark LC, Dalkin B, Krongrad A, et al. Decreased incidence of prostate cancer with selenium supplementation: Results of a double-blind cancer prevention trial. *Br J Urol* 1998; 81: 730-4.
37. Hofstad B, Almendingen K, Vatn M, et al. Growth and recurrence of colorectal polyps: A double-blind 3-year intervention with calcium and antioxidants. *Digestion* 1998; 59: 148-56.
38. Kinzler KW, Vogelstein B. Lessons from heredetary colorectal cancer. *Cell* 1996; 87: 159-70.
39. Muscat JE, Stellmann SD, Wynder EL. Nonsteroidal antiinflammatory drugs and colorectal cancer. *Cancer* 1994; 74: 1847-54.
40. Rosenberg L, Louik C, Shapiro S. Nonsteroidal antiinflammatory drug use and reduced risk of large bowel carcinoma. *Cancer* 1998; 82: 2326-33.

The adjuvant treatment of colon cancer

Eric Van Cutsem

Department of Internal Medicine, University Hospital Gasthuisberg, Leuven, Belgium

Colorectal cancer is most common in economically developed countries, particularly in parts of Europe, North America and Australia. The annual incidence varies between 55 and 0.7 per 100,000 people, respectively, in high- and low-risk populations. Colorectal cancer is one of the leading causes of cancer-related deaths in the Western world. Every year, colorectal cancer is responsible for an estimated 400,000 deaths worldwide. Approximately 60,000 people die from colorectal adenocarcinoma among the 150,000 new cases which are diagnosed in Europe each year.

Most patients (70%) who have colorectal cancer present with apparently localized disease. The remaining 30% have advanced disease at diagnosis, 25% of whom have distant metastatic disease and 5%, locally advanced disease. One quarter of colorectal cancer cases are confined to the rectum, while the remainder are located in some part of the colon.

Surgery is the only curative option for patients with colorectal cancer. Colorectal cancer is not uniformly fatal, although there are large differences in survival depending on stage of disease. Pathologic stage is presently the most important determinant of prognosis. The classification system described by Dukes in 1930 is still widely used. However, the original Dukes' system no longer fulfills the requirements of modern tumor staging, as it fails to take into account distant metastases, the number of lymph nodes involved, and carcinomas limited to the submucosa. Therefore the TNM classification of the American Joint Committee on Cancer (AJCC) is currently recommended for daily use and in clinical trials. The prognosis depends on the stage at which the tumor is diagnosed. In patients with a stage I tumor (pT1 or pT2N0M0), the 5-year survival amounts to > 90%. In patients with a stage II tumor (pT3 or pT4N0M0), the survival is variable. In patients with a pT3N0M0 tumor, the 5-year survival amounts to approximately 70%, while in patients with a pT4N0M0 tumor, the 5-year survival is much lower and is only around 30%. In patients with stage III tumors (pTXN+M0), the 5-year survival is 30-50%. In patients with metastatic colorectal cancer (stage IV), the 5-year survival is < 5% [1, 2].

Although the TNM classification is generally used to determine therapy for a given patient, other factors are thought to have an independent influence on outcome. Risk of recurrence appears to increase with bowel perforation, obstruction, the presence of venous, perineural or lymphatic invasion, poorly differentiation and elevated CEA level. More recently, it has been suggested that other factors might influence the recurrence rate and the prognosis of patients with resectable colon cancer, e.g.: DNA aneuploidy, the detection of micrometastases in lymph nodes by PCR, the thymidylate synthase level, overexpression of the *p53* gene, alterations in chromosome 18q (deleted in colon cancer - DCC- suppressor gene), and microsatellite instability (MSI) [3-8]. Although these factors and other new molecular factors can become extremely important in the future in the management of patients with colon cancer, neither of these factors are actually to be used systematically outside a clinical trial.

The adjuvant therapeutic modalities of colon and rectal cancer have to be differentiated. Rectal cancer can be defined as any tumor that is located either partly or entirely below the peritoneal reflection. This location makes it more difficult for surgeons to obtain wide margins at resection and is associated with a higher incidence of locoregional failure. Adjuvant therapies in patients with high-risk rectal cancer (stages II and III) must include an adequate surgical approach (Total Mesorectal Excision = TME) usually combined with a post- or preoperative radiotherapy, probably in combination with chemotherapy, to reduce the risk of local failure and of distant metastases and ultimately also to influence overall survival [7].

Adequate surgery by experienced surgeons is the basis of the treatment of resectable colon cancer and determines the prognosis. Surgery is the only curative option for patients with colorectal cancer. It has been shown too that the prognosis is also correlated with the number of detected and removed lymph nodes. An adjuvant therapy after surgery is administered with intent to target residual occult viable cells and eradicate them before they become established and relatively refractory to intervention. Important considerations are the risk-benefit ratio of such a treatment and the need to achieve a balance between maximum chance of cure/prolonged survival and tolerance or side effects.

Stage III colon cancer

The results of the adjuvant treatment in colon cancer are considered as one of the most important advances in clinical oncology over the last decade because of its impact and the implications of life savings, also due to frequency of colon cancer [1, 2].

The intergroup trial reported in 1990 by Moertel *et al.* (INT-0035) was the first large-scale study to demonstrate a significant survival benefit and a reduction in recurrence risk after postoperative treatment in patients with resected stage III colon cancer. This trial randomized 1,296 patients to one of three arms: (1) surgery alone, (2) surgery plus 12 months of levamisole, or (3) surgery plus 12 months of 5-fluorouracil (5-FU) plus levamisole. The study showed a 15% absolute reduction or ± 40% relative reduction in risk of recurrence and a 33% relative reduction in the overall death rate with the combination of surgery plus 5-FU/levamisole. Levamisole (LEV), a phenylimidothiazole compound, is an antihelminthic agent with immunomodulatory activity (T-cell stimulation), that has no effect on survival used alone adjuvantly [9, 10].

Since the combination of 5-FU and leucovorin (LV) has proved to be superior to 5-FU alone in patients with advanced colorectal cancer, a number of studies have confirmed the efficacy of 5-FU modulated by LV as adjuvant treatment, when compared with a no treatment control arm [11]. The NSABP (National Surgical Adjuvant Breast and Bowel project) protocol C-03 indicated a disease free (73% versus 64%) and overall (84% versus 77%) survival advantage for the 5-FU/LV combination when compared with MOF (methyl-CCNU, oncovin, 5-FU) at 3 years for patients with Dukes' stage B and C colon cancer [12]. The control arm in this study (MOF) had previously shown a survival advantage in the adjuvant setting. The Canadian and European consortium trial (IMPACT) compared adjuvant treatment with high-dose 5-FU and LV with no treatment in nearly 1500 patients; they demonstrated a 22% reduction in mortality at 3 years, both in Dukes' B and C patients [13]. A similar in design but smaller Italian study (Givio) showed a 39% reduction in mortality for the same group of patients [14]. With a median follow-up duration at 72 months, an intergroup study indicated that patients who received a combination of 5-FU and low dose LV over 6 months experienced significant improvement in time to relapse ($p < 0.01$) and survival ($p = 0.02$) compared with control patients treated with surgery alone. Based on indirect comparisons of the trials with 5-FU/levamisole and 5-FU/leucovorin, it was suggested therefore that both regimens were equally effective.

More recently the results of three large adjuvant American trials have been presented in which several thousands of patients have been treated. In a large, randomized study by the North Central Cancer Treatment Group (NCCTG) and the National Cancer Institute of Canada (NCIC), it was shown that there is no benefit associated with administration of a full year of chemotherapy compared with just 6 months of treatment with the same regimen [15]. In the same study, it is shown that, if only 6 months of chemotherapy was administered, patient survival was significantly inferior with the 5-FU plus levamisole regimen compared with the 3-drug 5-FU plus levamisole plus leucovorin regimen [15]. At the 1998 ASCO meeting, the intergroup reported moreover that there is no additional benefit from the addition of levamisole when 5-FU/leucovorin is given and that 6 months of treatment with 5-FU/leucovorin is as efficient as 12 months of 5-FU/levamisole (INT-0089) [16]. The NSABP C-04 study showed similar results *(table I)* [17]. Taking into account also the increased toxicity of the 3-drug combination (5-FU/leucovorin/levamisole) compared with the combination of 5-FU/leucovorin, it is accepted that a treatment with 5-FU/leucovorin for 6 months is nowadays the standard treatment in Dukes'C colon carcinoma [18, 19].

Two regimens of 5 FU/LV are proposed in the USA: weekly LV (500 mg/m^2) plus 5-FU (500 mg/m^2) during 6 weeks followed by 2 weeks of rest or the "Mayo Clinic Regimen": LV (20 mg/m^2) + 5-FU (425 mg/m^2) d. 1-5 repeated every 4 weeks. In Europe the Mayo Clinic Regimen is usually proposed as the standard regimen. Several new ongoing studies are evaluating the role of other 5-FU/LV regimens in the adjuvant treatment: infusional 5-FU, infusional 5-FU/LV and shorter duration (3 months). It has indeed been shown that infusional 5-FU/LV regimens are more efficient in terms of response rate and time to tumor progression (TTP) than bolus 5-FU/LV regimens in patients with advanced colorectal cancer [20]. Despite greater technical requirements, the tolerance of infusional 5-FU

Table I. Results of three large adjuvant American trials.

Trial	Regimen	N° of patients	5-year disease-free survival rate (%)	5-year overall survival rate (%)
NCCTG-NCIC [15]	5-FU/levamisole (6 mo)	230	58	60
	5-FU/folinic acid (Mayo Clinic regimen) + levamisole (6 mo)	225	63	70
	5-FU/levamisole (1 yr)	228	63	68
	5-FU/folinic acid (Mayo Clinic regimen) + levamisole (1 yr)	232	57	63
INT 0089 [16]	5-FU/levamisole (1 yr)	833	56	63
	5-FU/folinic acid weekly (8 mo)	946	59	65
	5-FU/folinic acid (Mayo Clinic regimen) (6 mo)	953	60	66
	5-FU/folinic acid (Mayo Clinic regimen) + levamisole (6 mo)	827	60	67
NSABP C-04 [17]	5-FU/levamisole (1 yr)	691	60	70
	5-FU/folinic acid weekly (1 yr)	691	65	74
	5-FU/folinic acid weekly + levamisole (1 yr)	696	64	73

5-FU = Fluorouracil; NCCTG = North Central Cancer Treatment Group; NCIC = National Cancer Institute of Canada; INT = Intergroup; NSABP = National Surgical Adjuvant Breast and Bowel Project.

regimens was better than of bolus regimens in patients with advanced colorectal cancer. Preliminary results of two studies have shown the feasibility of infusional regimens and a different toxicity pattern compared to bolus regimens in the adjuvant treatment of colon cancer. These preliminary results showed an identical disease free survival and median survival [21, 22].

Stage II colon cancer

The question whether stage II or Dukes' B2 cancer patients should be treated with an adjuvant chemotherapy remains controversial in 2000. Most of the published trials on the adjuvant treatment of colon cancer include as well stage II as stage III colon cancer. Data from large prospective trials in stage II colon cancer alone that allow to draw definitive conclusions on the role of adjuvant treatment in this setting are still lacking. The INT-0035 trial, which compared 5-FU plus levamisole with surgery alone, showed a similar reduction in the rate of recurrence (32%) in stage II as was observed in stage III cancer. No benefit in overall survival was shown, probably because of the relative lack of power of this study [9, 10].

The International Multicentre Pooled Analysis of B2 Colon Cancer Trials (IMPACT B2) investigators, after combining five separate trials in which patients were randomized to postoperative fluorouracil and folinic acid (FU + LV) or to no further therapy, conclude, that their analysis does not support the routine use of FU + LV in all patients with B2 colon cancer. The 5-year overall survival was 80% and 82% and the event-free survival 73% and 76% resp. for controls and for 5-FU/leucovorin treated patients [23].

However, the National Surgical Adjuvant Breast and Bowel Project (NSABP) group, after combining data from four of the group's trials including stage B and C colon cancer patients, reports that patients with Dukes'B colon cancer benefit from adjuvant chemotherapy. The relative reduction in mortality, recurrence or disease-free survival event was in most instances of the NSABP trials as great or greater for Dukes' B patients than for Dukes' C patients. The mortality reduction was 30% for Dukes' B patients and this occurred irrespective of the presence of absence of adverse prognostic factors [24].

Therefore probably only a subgroup of stage II patients really benefits from postoperative treatment [18, 19, 25, 26]. The value of molecular prognostic factors such as aneuploidy, expression of p53 or p21, microsatellite instability (MSI), overexpression of thymidylate synthase, and absence of expression of the deleted-in-colorectal cancer gene (DCC) are currently under investigation for stratifying patients for an adjuvant treatment. Clinical and pathologic prognostic factors such as young age, perforation or occlusion as presenting symptom, and the presence of perineural, venous or lymphatic invasion can currently be used to identify patients at higher risk for recurrence and to select stage II patients for an adjuvant treatment outside of a clinical trial.

Portal vein infusion and intraperitoneal chemotherapy

Several randomised trials have been performed to study the effect of an intraportal infusion of 5-FU, administered immediately after the operation. The rationale of this treatment was that colorectal cancer recurrences are often seen in the liver. Initially a number of positive results have been reported. These could, however, not always be confirmed. A meta-analysis of 9 trials of adjuvant postoperative intraportal chemotherapy was performed. A small but significant benefit in survival was found: the reduction in death was 13% [27]. However it cannot be explained why the incidence of liver metastases was not lower. This suggests a systemic effect of intraportal chemotherapy that could be possibly attributed to the early postoperative administration of chemotherapy. In contrast, a more recent well performed large randomised EORTC trial could not show an effect of intraportal adjuvant chemotherapy [28]. We can therefore conclude that intraportal chemotherapy is an interesting concept, but that the systematic use in clinical practice should not be advised.

Another interesting technique currently under investigation in the adjuvant treatment of colorectal cancer is **intraperitoneal chemotherapy**, in combination with systemic treatment. Such an approach would have the potential advantage of acting on both microscopic peritoneal tumor spread as well as on liver micrometastases, since intraperitoneal 5-FU is absorbed through the portal vein and results in a high 5-FU concentration in the portal blood. Although the benefit of such an approach is not proven, a small randomised study from investigators in Austria indicates a possible advantage over conventional adjuvant therapy. Patients with resected Dukes' B or C colon cancer were assigned to either intravenous and intraperitoneal 5-FU/LV or intravenous 5-FU/LEV as the "standard therapy" arm. A preliminary analysis after a median follow-up time of 27 months showed a significant disease free survival advantage in favor of the experimental arm (17/94 versus 35/96 recurrences, p = 0.0015) [29].

The EORTC performed a 4-arm trial to study the role of postoperative regional chemotherapy in association with systemic chemotherapy (6 months 5-FU/leucovorin versus 5-FU/levamisole). Results are not yet available.

Immunotherapy

A growing interest in the immunological treatments of malignancy has led to the development of both specific and non-specific immunotherapy adjuvant trials in colorectal cancer. One of the first studies (NSABP C-01) had a three arm randomisation to either no postoperative therapy, MOF chemotherapy, or intradermal BCG. At 5 years' follow-up, the BCG treatment group demonstrated a slight survival advantage compared with surgery alone, although there was no difference in terms of disease free survival in the two groups [30].

The concept of using vaccines to induce specific immunity against carcinomas has been actively pursued over the last two decades. Early attempts to induce tumor regression in cancer patients by inducing tumor-specific immunity with autologous or allogeneic tumor cell vaccines were not successful. A European trial showed a longer recurrence-free period and a risk reduction for recurrence but no survival advantage for active specific immunotherapy (ASI) with an autologous tumor cell-BCG vaccine in the adjuvant treatment of stage II colon cancer [31]. An American trial, however, did not show a clinical benefit in patients with stage II and III colon cancer [32].

Another direction of immunotherapy is the development of monoclonal antibodies. The murine monoclonal antibody against the 17-1A antigen, Panorex, has been shown in a small randomised study to reduce the mortality with 32% and the relapse rate with 23% at a median follow-up of 7 years in Dukes' C colorectal cancer [33]. This monoclonal antibody plus 5-FU/LV is now being compared with 5-FU/LV alone in two large scale randomised phase 3 studies in stage III colon cancer. In stage II colon cancer, a randomised trial of this monoclonal antibody after surgery versus surgery alone is ongoing (CALGB-EORTC).

New drugs

The role of the oral fluoropyrimidines, capecitabine and UFT (uracil and tegafur) in the adjuvant treatment of colon cancer is currently under investigation in large scale randomised phase III studies.

The topoisomerase I inhibitor irinotecan (CPT-11) and the diaminocyclohexane platinum derivative, oxaliplatin, are two new active drugs in advanced colon cancer and hold promise as potentially effective drugs in early colon cancer. Large phase III trials are at present ongoing to evaluate the role of irinotecan in association with 5-FU/LV and of oxaliplatin also in combination with 5-FU/LV in the adjuvant treatment of stage II and III colon cancer.

References

1. Moore HCF, Haller DG. Adjuvant therapy of colon cancer. *Semin Oncol* 1999; 26: 545-55.
2. Saltz LB, Kemeny NE. Adjuvant chemotherapy of colorectal cancer. *The Oncologist* 1996; 1: 22-9.
3. Liefers GJ, Cleton-Jansen AM, van de Velde CJ, Hermans J, van Krieken JH, Cornelisse CJ, Tollenaar RA. Micrometastases and survival in stage II colorectal cancer. *N Engl J Med* 1998; 339: 223-8.
4. Gryfe R, Kim H, Hsieh ETK, Aronson MD, Holowaty EJ, Bull SB, Redston M, Gallinger S. Tumor microsatellite instability and clinical outcome in young patients with colorectal cancer. *N Engl J Med* 2000; 342: 69-77.
5. Jernvall P, Mäkinen MJ, Karttunen TJ, Mäkelä J, Vihko P. Microsatellite instability: Impact on cancer progression in proximal and distal colorectal cancers. *Eur J Cancer* 1999; 35: 197-201.
6. Bouzourene H, Gervaz P, Cerottini JP, Benhattar J, Chaubert P, Saraga E, Pampallona S, Bosman FT, Givel JC. p53 and Ki-ras as prognostic factors for Dukes' stage B colorectal cancer. *Eur J Cancer* 2000; 36: 1008-15.
7. Van Cutsem E, Peeters M, Verslype C, Filez L, Haustermans K, Janssens J. The medical treatment of colorectal cancer: Actual status and new developments. *Hepato-Gastroenterology* 1999; 46: 709-16.
8. Elsaleh H, Joseph D, Grieu F, Zeps N, Spry N, Lacopetta B. Association of tumour site and sex with survival benefit from adjuvant chemotherapy in colorectal cancer. *Lancet* 2000; 355: 1745-50.
9. Moertel CG, Fleming TR, Macdonald JS, Haller DG, Laurie JA, Goodman PJ, Ungerleider JS, Emerson WA, Tormey DC, Glick JH. Levamisole and fluorouracil for adjuvant therapy of resected colon carcinoma. *N Engl J Med* 1990; 322: 352-8.
10. Moertel CG, Fleming TR, Macdonald JS, Haller DG, Laurie JA, Tangen CM, Ungerleider JS, Emerson WA, Tormey DC, Glick JH, Veeder MH, Mailliard JA for the North Central Cancer Treatment group, Southwest Oncology Group, and Eastern Cooperative Oncology Group. Intergroup study of fluorouracil plus levamisole as adjuvant therapy for stage II/Dukes' B2 colon cancer. *J Clin Oncol* 1995; 13: 2936-43.
11. Advanced Colorectal Cancer Meta-Analysis Project: Modulation of fluorouracil by leucovorin in patients with advanced colorectal cancer: Evidence in terms of response rate. *J Clin Oncol* 1992; 10: 896-903.
12. Wolmark N, Rockette H, Fisher B, Wickerham DL, Redmond C, Fisher ER, Jones J, Mamounas EP, Ore L, Petrelli NJ. The benefit of leucovorin-modulated fluorouracil as postoperative adjuvant therapy for primary colon cancer: Results from National Surgical Adjuvant Breast and Bowel Project protocol C-03. *J Clin Oncol* 1993; 11: 1879-87.
13. International Multicentre Pooled Analysis of Colorectal Cancer Trials (IMPACT). Efficacy of adjuvant fluorouracil and folinic acid in colon cancer. *Lancet* 1995; 345: 939-44.
14. Francini G, Petrioli R, Lorenzini L, Mancini S, Armenio S, Tanzini G, Marsili S, Aquino A, Marzocca G, Civitelli S. Folinic acid and 5-fluorouracil as adjuvant chemotherapy in colon cancer. *Gastroenterology* 1994; 106: 899-906.

15. O'Connell MJ, Laurie JA, Kahn M, Fitzgibbons RJ Jr, Erlichman C, Shepherd L, Moertel CG, Kocha WI, Pazdur R, Wieand HS, Rubin J, Vukov AM, Donohue JH, Krook JE, Figueredo A. Prospectively randomized trial of postoperative adjuvant chemotherapy in patients with high-risk colon cancer. *J Clin Oncol* 1998; 16: 295-300.
16. Haller D, Catalano P, MacDonald J, Mayer R. Fluorouracil (FU), leucovorin (LV) and levamisole (LEV) adjuvant therapy for colon cancer: Five-year final report of INT-0089 (abstract). *Proc Am Soc Clin Oncol* 1998; 17: 256a.
17. Wolmark N, Rockette H, Mamounas E, Jones J, Wieand S, Wickerham DL, Bear HD, Atkins JN, Dimitrov NV, Glass AG, Fisher ER, Fisher B. Clinical trial to assess the relative efficacy of fluorouracil and leucovorin, fluorouracil and levamisole and fluorouracil, leucovorin and levamisole in patients with Dukes' B and C carcinoma of the colon: results from National Surgical Adjuvant Breast and Bowel Project C-04. *J Clin Oncol* 1999; 17: 3553-9.
18. Michel P, Merle V, Chiron A, Ducrotte P, Paillot B, Hecketsweiler P, Czernichow P, Colin R. Postoperative management of stage II/III colon cancer: A decision analysis. *Gastroenterology* 1999; 117: 784-93.
19. Slevin ML, Papamichael D, Rougier P, Schmoll HJ. Current controversies in cancer. Is there a standard adjuvant treatment for colon cancer? *Eur J Cancer* 1998; 34: 1652-63.
20. Van Cutsem E, Peeters M. Developments in fluoropyrimidine therapy for gastrointestinal cancer. *Eur Opin Oncol* 1999; 11: 312-7.
21. Saini A, Cunningham D, Norman AR, Hill ME, Tait D, Hickish T, Iveson T, Lofts F, Jodrell D, Ross PJ, Oates JR. Multicentre randomized trial of protracted venous infusion (PVI) 5 FU compared to 5 FU/folinic acid (5FU/FA) as adjuvant therapy for colorectal cancer. *Proc Am Soc Clin Oncol* 2000; 19: 240a.
22. Poplin E, Benedetti J, Estes N, Haller D, Mayer R, Goldberg R, Macdonald J. Phase III randomized trial of bolus 5-FU/Leucovorin/Levamisole versus 5-FU continuous infusion/levamisole as adjuvant therapy for high risk colon cancer (SWOG 9415/INT-0153). *Proc Am Soc Clin Oncol* 2000; 19: 240a.
23. International Multicentre Pooled Analysis of BS Colon Cancer Trials (IMPACT B2) Investigators. Efficacy of adjuvant fluorouracil and folinic acid in B2 colon cancer. *J Clin Oncol* 1999; 17: 1356-63.
24. Mamounas E, Wieand S, Wolmark N, Bear HD, Atkins JN, Song K, Jones J, Rockette H. Comparative efficacy of adjuvant chemotherapy in patients with Dukes' B versus Dukes' C colon cancer: Results from four national surgical adjuvant breast and bowel project adjuvant studies (C-01, C-02, C-03, and C-04). *J Clin Oncol* 1999; 17: 1349-55.
25. Harrington DP. The tea leaves of small trials. *J Clin Oncol* 1999; 17: 1336-8.
26. Schrag D. Defining optimal treatment for stage II colon cancer: Does decision analysis help? *Gastroenterology* 1999; 117: 1005-8.
27. Liver infusion meta-analysis group. Portal vein chemotherapy for colorectal cancer: A meta-analysis of 4000 patients in 10 studies. *J Natl Cancer Inst* 1997; 89: 497-505.
28. Rougier P, Sahmoud T, Nitti D, Curran D, Doci R, De Waele B, Nakajima T, Rauschecker H, Labianca R, Pector J-C, Marsoni S, Apolone G, Lasser P, Couvreur ML, Wils J, the European Organisation for Research and Treatment of Cancer Gastrointestinal Tract Cancer Cooperative Group, the Gruppo Interdisciplinare Valutazione Interventi in Oncologia, and the Japanese Foundation for Cancer Research. Adjuvant portal-vein infusion of fluorouracil and heparin in colorectal cancer: a randomised trial. *Lancet* 1998; 351: 1677-81.
29. Scheithauer W, Kornek GV, Marczell A, Karner J, Salem G, Greiner R, Burger D, Stöger F, Ritschel J Kovats E, Vischer HM, Schneeweiss B, Depisch D. Combined intravenous and intraperitoneal chemotherapy with fluorouracil + leucovorin vs fluorouracil + levamisole for adjuvant therapy of resected colon carcinoma. *Brit J Cancer* 1998; 77: 1349-54.

30. Wolmark N, Fisher B, Rockette H, Redmond C, Wickerham DL, Fisher ER, Jones J, Glass A, Lerner H, Lawrence W. Postoperative adjuvant chemotherapy or BCG for colon cancer: results from NSABP protocol C-01. *J Natl Cancer Inst* 1988; 80: 30-6.
31. Vermorken JB, Claessen AME, van Tinteren H, Gall HE, Ezinga R, Meijer S, Scheper RJ, Meijer CJLM, Bloemena E, Ransom JH, Hanna Jr MG, Pinedo HM. Active specific immunotherapy for stage II and stage III human colon cancer: a randomised trial. *Lancet* 1999; 353: 345-50.
32. Harris JE, Ryan L, Hoover Jr HC, Stuart RK, Oken MM, Benson III AB, Mansour E, Haller DG, Manola J, Hanna Jr MG. Adjuvant active specific immunotherapy for stage II and III colon cancer with an autologous tumor cell vaccine: Eastern Cooperative Oncology Group Study E5283. *J Clin Oncol* 2000; 18: 148-57.
33. Riethmüller G, Holz E, Schlimok G, Schmiegel W, Raab R, Höffken K, Gruber R, Funke I, Pichlmaier H, Hirche H, Buggisch P, Witte J, Pichlmayr R. Monoclonal antibody therapy for resected Dukes' C colorectal cancer: Seven-year outcome of a multicenter randomized trial. *J Clin Oncol* 1998; 16: 1788-94.

individual patient the expected benefits have to be weighted against the possible toxicities of treatment.

5-fluorouracil (5-FU)

The antimetabolite 5-fluorouracil (5-FU) has been the cornerstone of palliative drug treatment for more than 40 years. However, the response rate to this drug when applied as a single agent is poor (10-15%) and the many clinical trials performed have failed to show a major impact on survival. Efforts have been made to improve the efficacy of 5-FU by different approaches: biochemical modulation with leucovorin, methotrexate or (α-interferon; combinations of 5-FU with other cytotoxic agents; and changes in the schedule of administration. In a meta-analysis of nine randomised clinical trials comparing 5-FU/LV with 5-FU alone, a significantly higher response rate of 23% (range, 16-48%; 803 patients) was achieved with the combination compared with 11% (range, 7- 17%; 578 patients) observed with 5-FU alone [1]. There was, however, no significant benefit in terms of prolonged survival. One possible explanation for the latter is that many patients not responding crossed over from 5-FU alone to 5-FU/LV, thus potentially masking any survival disadvantage of single treatment 5-FU. Alternatively, it may be that this observation reflects the only modest advantage of 5-FU/LV over 5-FU alone. Other concerns center around the optimal treatment regimen; weekly *versus* monthly (daily, on five consecutive days) treatment intervals, and the dose of leucovorin; high *versus* low dose. The analyzed trials show similar response rates for the weekly and monthly schedules. Only with the weekly regimens it seems that the dose of leucovorin is important, the high dose showing a higher response rate. A further important factor is the mode of administration. Protracted venous infusion of 5-FU (PVI 5-FU) has the theoretical advantage of exposing increased numbers of malignant cells in the S-phase of the cell cycle to the drug (5-FU is a S-phase specific drug) and it permits the delivery of higher cumulative doses. A recent meta-analysis of six randomised trials including 1,219 patients comparing 5-FU bolus with PVI-5-FU, showed PVI-5-FU to be superior in terms of response (22% *vs* 14%) [2]. However, again only a slight increase of overall survival accompanied the increased response rates. In summary, it appears that regardless of which schedule of 5-FU administration is used, a large proportion of patients with metastatic colorectal cancer does not respond to this therapy.

An exciting prospect is the development of oral compounds based on 5-FU. These include S-1, capecitabine, UFT (ftorafur with uracil), and ethynyluracil combined with 5-FU. Most of these drugs incorporate inhibitors of the enzyme dihydropyrimidine dehydrogenase which produces a significant decrease in 5-FU catabolism thereby providing prolonged elevated plasma levels of 5-FU and mimicking continuous infusion therapy.

Irinotecan

The recent introduction of the camptothecin CPT-11 (irinotecan), a topoisomerase I inhibitor, was an important breakthrough in the treatment of colorectal cancer. The main mechanism of action of camptothecins is the stabilization of the DNA-topoisomerase I complex upon processing of the replication fork, causing single- and double-strand DNA breaks, thereby inhibiting transcription and DNA replication which ultimately result in cell death. The two schedules most often used in phase II and III trials in colorectal cancer are i.v. bolus administration of CPT-11 at a dose of 350 mg/m^2 every 3 weeks, and 125 mg/m^2 once a week for 4 weeks followed by two weeks rest. The most important toxicities are neutropenia and diarrhea. Phase II studies in chemo-naive patients with colorectal cancer showed response rates of 20-30%. An important observation made in phase II studies was the finding of comparable response rates in chemotherapy-naive, 5-FU pretreated, and 5-FU refractory patients suggesting a lack of cross-resistance and that patients unresponsive to 5-FU may still benefit from CPT-11. Two randomised trials, comparing CPT-11 with continuous infusion 5-FU and supportive care alone in patients with failure on 5-FU, showed superiority for CPT-11 with respect to survival and quality of life *(table I)* [3, 4]. However, the observed survival benefit was small (2 to 3 months) and has to be weighed against the side-effects and costs of the drug. Based on these studies, CPT-11 seemed a reasonable option for second-line treatment in patients with good performance status and progressive metastatic colorectal cancer. Recently two studies addressing CPT-11 in the first-line treatment of advanced colorectal cancer have been presented *(table II)* [5, 6].

Table I. CPT-11 in 5-FU resistant or refractory patients.

Author	N° of patients	Treatment	Progression free survival (months)	Overall survival (months)
Cunningham et al. [4]	279	CPT-11 300/350 mg/m^2 vs Supportive care	-	9.2 6.5
Rougier et al. [3]	267	CPT-11 300/350 mg/m^2 vs 5-FU c.i. (plus LV)	4.2 2.9	8.5 10.8

Table II. First-line CPT-11/5-FU/LV in colorectal cancer.

Author	N° of patients	Treatment	Response rate	Time to progression (months)	Overall survival (months)
Douillard et al. [5]	387	CPT-11+5-FU/LV vs 5-FU/LV	35% 22%	6.7 4.4	17.4 14.1
Saltz et al. [6]	667	CPT-11+5-FU/LV vs 5-FU/LV vs CPT-11	39% 21% 18%	7.0 4.3 4.2	14.8 12.6 12.0

Combination treatment with CPT-11 plus 5-FU resulted in significantly higher response rates compared to 5-FU or CPT-11 alone, 35% *versus* 20%. However, this significant increased response rate is poorly reflected in the progression free and overall survival which were prolonged with only a few months. An explanation for the latter is that the studies allowed the control arm to receive second-line chemotherapy, mostly CPT-11.

Toxicities observed were acceptable, with more diarrhea and neutropenia in the CPT-11/5-FU/LV group compared to the 5-FU/LV only group. And quality of life evaluation was also in favor of the combined treatment. Based on these studies it seems reasonable to offer patients first-line combination treatment with CPT-11/5-FU/LV, especially when the patients have a good performance score, minimal disease, and if surgery is an option in case of response. An important question which remains to be answered is: is first-line combination chemotherapy with 5-FU and CPT-11 better than sequential treatment?

Oxaliplatin

Single-agent oxaliplatin, a third generation platinum analogue, showed response rates of 10% in advanced colorectal cancer. When combined with high dose leucovorin and continuous infusion of 5-FU in phase II studies response rates up to 50-60% are reported, even in patients resistant to 5-FU/LV. Best results were obtained with chronomodulation, which means adjustment of the dosing time of chemotherapy to the natural circadian rhythm. Despite these figures, the lack of phase III studies comparing oxaliplatin to 5-FU/LV and the complexity of chronomodulation were reasons for skepticism by many. However, recent phase III studies in untreated patients showed a significant improved response rate when oxaliplatin was added to 5-FU/LV. The first study showed an increase in response rate from 16% to 53% when oxaliplatin was added to a schedule of chronomodulated 5-FU/LV and progression free survival was prolonged with 3 months *(table III)* [7]. Another phase III study compared flat rate 5-FU/LV with oxaliplatin/5-FU/LV and showed an increased response rate and progression free survival for the combination group compared to the 5-FU/LV only group, 50.7 vs 22.3% and 9.0 vs 6.2 months, respectively [8]. Despite this high response rate and a significant prolonged progression free survival there was no significant prolongation of the overall survival. Cross-over and post-study second-line treatment (irinotecan or oxaliplatin) of patients in the control-arm seems the cause. The most important side-effects observed were a reversible peripheral sensitive neuropathy, neutropenia and diarrhea. Quality of life scores were equal for both arms. In a randomised study comparing constant rate infusion with chronotherapy of the combination oxaliplatin, leucovorin and 5-FU, response rates of 51% and 21% respectively were observed. Based on these results oxaliplatin is accepted for first-line treatment of colorectal cancer.

Table III. First-line oxaliplatin/5-FU/LV in colorectal cancer.

Author	N° of patients	Treatment	Response rate	Progression free survival (months)	Overall survival (months)
Giachetti et al. [7]	200	5 d 5-FU/LV+oxaliplatin 5 d 5-FU/LV	53% 16%	8.7 6.1	19.9 19.4
De Gramont et al. [8]	420	c.i. 5-FU/LV+oxaliplatin vs. c.i. 5-FU/LV	51% 22%	9.0 6.2 (P=0.0003)	16.2 14.7 (P0.12)

Therapeutic choices in colorectal cancer

With the introduction of new active drugs, such as CPT-11 and oxaliplatin, therapeutic choices have to be made. At this moment the best therapy in colorectal cancer is not known. A possible approach is the use of predictive factors. By the use of predictive factors, such as thymidylate synthase (TS) and dihydropyrimidine dehydrogenase (DPD), it is possible to select patients who are likely to respond to a 5-FU-based treatment and to exclude patients who will not respond. With low TS and low DPD predicting for response to 5-FU and high TS and/or high DPD predicting for resistance to 5-FU [9-11]. The major advantage of such an approach will be that patients will not be exposed unnecessarily to a possibly toxic treatment and can immediately receive TS and DPD independent regimens in first-line. CPT-11 and oxaliplatin are both TS independent drugs, have a different mechanism of action and showed synergistic activity *in vitro*. The drugs show no overlapping toxicities. Furthermore, the combination CPT-11/oxaliplatin showed considerable efficacy in the treatment of metastatic colorectal cancer with response rates of 42% reported in 5-FU/LV pretreated patients. At our institute we are doing a study in patients with advanced colorectal cancer in which the first-line treatment of patients with advanced colorectal cancer will be TS and DPD dependent chemotherapy (5-FU/LV), or TS and DPD independent chemotherapy (CPT-11/oxaliplatin). Treatment choice will be based on TS and DPD determination in biopsy specimens of tumor tissue *(figure 1)*.

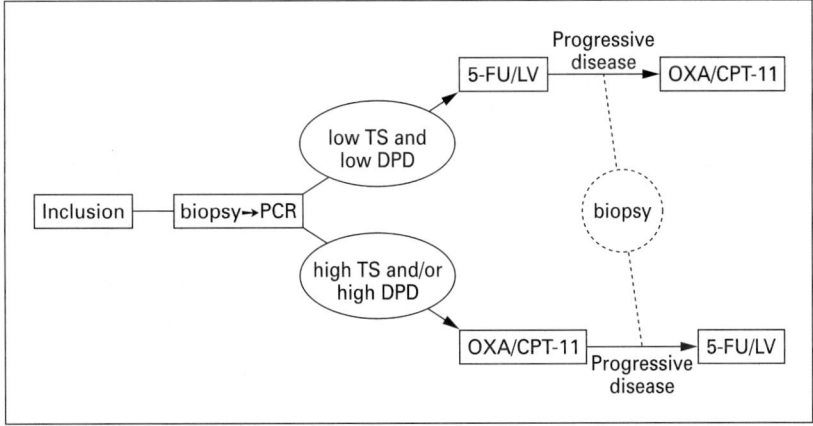

Figure 1. Treatment choice based on TS and DPD determination in biopsy specimens of tumor tissue.

Hepatic arterial chemotherapy

The liver is an important site of metastatic disease in colorectal cancer. About 60% of patients will develop liver metastases, and the liver is the only metastatic site in as many as 30-40% of patients with advanced disease. The presence of hepatic metastases has a major impact on survival with reported 1- and 3-year survival rates in untreated patients of 31% and 2.6%, respectively. If disease is confined to the liver, and surgery is not an option, liver directed therapy is a logical approach. The principal advantage of hepatic arterial chemotherapy is the possibility to achieve higher drug concentrations at the tumor site compared to systemic treatment, while reducing systemic exposure and hence, toxicity. Liver metastases derive their blood supply from the hepatic artery, while normal hepatocytes derive most of their blood supply from the portal vein. When chemotherapy is administered intravenously, only a fraction of the drug reaches the liver, whereas administration into the hepatic artery results in increased local drug concentrations, thereby exposing the metastatic tumor cells to higher drug levels. This regional advantage will be further increased in case of a high total body clearance of the drug. Moreover, high first-pass hepatic extraction of the drug will result in high local concentrations with low systemic exposure allowing the delivery of higher doses of drugs [12]. 5-FU and fluorodeoxyuridine (FUDR) are the drugs most commonly used in hepatic arterial infusion chemotherapy for liver metastases of colorectal cancer. Randomised trials comparing HAC with systemic treatment or best supportive care [13-18] showed a clear benefit for HAC with respect to tumor response; however, a significant prolongation of survival with HAC was not demonstrated in most studies *(table IV)*. A meta-analysis comprising 654 patients showed objective response rates were 41% in patients treated with HAC and 14% in patients receiving intravenous chemotherapy [19]. Disappointingly, still no clinical significant survival advantage for HAC over systemic treatment was substantiated (16 months *versus* 12.2 months, p = 0.14). On the other hand, both studies comparing HAC to an *ad libitum* control group showed a significant prolonged survival for HAC (14.5 months *versus* 10.1 months, p = 0.002). The latter might be explained by cross-over, technical

Table IV. Randomised trials comparing hepatic arterial chemotherapy (HAC) with systemic treatment.

Author	N° of patients HAC/control[1]	HAC treatment	Control group	Response rate HAC vs control	Median survival (in months) HAC vs control
Kemeny [13] (1987)	48(45)/ 51(48)	FUDR 0.3 mg/kg/day (14 days every 28 days)	FUDR 0.15 mg/kg/day i.v. (14 days every 28 days)	50% vs 19.6% (P=0.001)	17 vs 12 (P=0.42)
Rougier [14] (1992)	81(70)/ 82(41)	FUDR 0.3 mg/kg/day (14 days every 28 days)	5-FU bolus i.v. 500 mg/m² (5 days every 28 days) or no chemotherapy (41pt.)	43% vs 9%[2]	15 vs 11 (P<0.02)
Martin [15] (1990)	36(31)/ 33(33)	FUDR 0.3 mg/kg/day (14 days every 28 days)	5-FU bolus i.v. 500 mg/m² (5 days every 35 days)	48% vs 21% (P=0.02)	12.6 vs 10.5 (P=0.53)
Hohn [17] (1989)	67(50)/ 76(65)	FUDR 0.3 mg/kg/day After 25 pt 0.2 mg/kg/day (14 days every 28 days)	FUDR 0.075 mg/kg/day[3] i.v. (14 days every 28 days)	42% vs 10% (P=0.0001)	16.6 vs 16 (P=N.S.)
Allen-Mersh [16] (1994)	51(49)/ 49(10)	FUDR 0.2 mg/kg/day (14 days every 28 days)	Symptom control only or *ad libitum* chemotherapy (10 pt.)	40%	13.4 vs 7.5 (P=0.03)
Chang [18] (1987)	32(21)/ 32(29)	FUDR 0.3 mg/kg/day (14 days every 28 days)	FUDR 0.125 mg/kg/day (14 days every 28 days)	62% vs 17% (P=0.003)	7 vs 12 (P=0.27)

[1] Patients randomised to HAC or i.v. treatment and ( ) patients actually receiving therapy; [2] patients who received i.v. chemotherapy; [3] intercycle escalation with 0,025 mg/kg/day depending on occurring toxicity.

difficulties related to delivery of the drug and progression of disease outside the liver. Based on these results hepatic, arterial chemotherapy cannot be regarded as a standard treatment option and should be given in clinical trials only.

Conclusions and future aspects

During the past decade, the development of new cytostatic drugs has increased the therapeutic options in colorectal cancer. However, many issues remain unresolved and new questions have a risen. The most important are: What is the optimal first-line treatment of advanced colorectal cancer? Why are the higher response rates not translated in a more prolonged survival? And, what is the reason for the low rate of complete responses observed?

Furthermore, new treatment modalities, such as immunotherapy, genetherapy and anti-angiogenetic drugs are under development. Studies with new combination treatments, the possible role of predictive factors, and new treatment modalities are needed in order to develop an effective treatment strategy in patients with advanced colorectal cancer.

References

1. Project BtACCM-A. Modulation of fluorouracil by leucovorin in patients with advanced colorectal cancer: evidence in terms of response rate. *J Clin Oncol* 1992; 10: 896-903.
2. Cancer BtM-aGi. Efficacy of intravenous continuous infusion of fluorouracil compared with bolus administration in advanced colorectal cancer. *J Clin Oncol* 1998; 16: 301-8.
3. Rougier P, Cutsem Ev, Bajetta E, et al Randomised trial of irinotecan versus fluorouracil by continuous infusion after fluorouracil failure in patients with metastatic colorectal cancer. *Lancet* 1998; 352: 1407-12.
4. Cunningham D, Pyrhonen S, James RD, et al. Randomised trial of irinotecan plus supportive care versus supportive care alone after fluorouracil failure for patients with metastatic colorectal cancer. *Lancet* 1998; 352: 1423-8.
5. Douillard JY, Cunningham D, Roth AD, et al. Irinotecan combined with fluorouracil compared with fluorouracil alone as first-line treatment for metastatic colorectal cancer: a multicentre randomised trial. *Lancet* 2000; 355: 1041-7.
6. Saltz LB, Locker PK, Pirotta N, et al. Weekly irinotecan (CPT-11), leucovorin (LV), and fluorouracil (FU) is superior to daily x5 LV/FU in patients (pts) with previously untreated metastatic colorectal cancer (CRC), Proceedings of the American Society of Clinical Oncology. Atlanta, 1999: 898.
7. Giachetti S, Perpoint B, Zidani R, et al. Phase III multicenter randomized trial of oxaliplatin added to the chronomodulated fluorouracil-leucovorin as first-line treatment of metastatic colorectal cancer. *J Clin Oncol* 2000; 18: 136-47.
8. Gramont Ad, Figer A, Seymour M, et al. Leucovorin and fluorouracil with or without oxaliplatin as first-line treatment in advanced colorectal cancer. *J Clin Oncol* 2000; 18: 2938-47.
9. Danenberg K, Metzger R, Groshen S, et al. Thymidylate synthase (TS) and thymidine phosphorylase (TP) are prognostic indicators of survival for colorectal cancer., Proceedings American Society of Clinical Oncology, 1997: A257.

10. Leichman CG, Lenz HJ, Leichman L, *et al.* Quantitation of intratumoral thymidylate synthase expression predicts for disseminated colorectal cancer response to protracted-infusion fluorouracil and weekly leucovorin. *J Clin Oncol* 1997; 15: 3223-9.
11. Peters GJ, Wilt CLvd, Groeningen CJv, *et al.* Thymidylate synthase inhibition after administration of fluorouracil with or without leucovorin in colon cancer patients: implications for treatment with fluorouracil. *J Clin Oncol* 1994; 12: 2035-42.
12. Ensminger WD, Gyves JW: Clinical pharmacology of hepatic arterial chemotherapy. *Semin Oncol* 1983; 10: 176-82.
13. Kemeny N, Daly J, Reichman B, *et al.* Intrahepatic or systemic infusion of fluorodeoxyuridine in patients with liver metastases from colorectal carcinoma. *Ann Intern Med* 1987; 107: 459-65.
14. Rougier P, Laplanche A, Huguier M, *et al.* Hepatic arterial infusion of floxuridine in patients with liver metastases from colorectal carcinoma: long-term results of a prospective randomized trial. *J Clin Oncol* 1992; 10: 1112-8.
15. Martin JK, O'Connel MJ, Wieand HS, *et al.* Intra-arterial floxuridine vs systemic fluorouracil for hepatic metastases from colorectal cancer. *Arch Surg* 1990; 125: 1022-7.
16. Allen-Mersh TG, Earlam S, Fordy C, *et al.* Quality of life and survival with continuous hepatic-artery floxuridine infusion for colorectal liver metastases. *Lancet* 1994; 344: 1255-60.
17. Hohn DC, Stagg RJ, Friedman MA, *et al.* A randomized trial of continuous intravenous versus hepatic intraarterial floxuridine in patients with colorectal cancer metastatic to the liver: The Northern California Oncology Group Trial. *J Clin Onco* 1989; 7: 1646-54.
18. Chang AE, Schneider PD, Sugarbaker PH, *et al.* A prospective randomized trial of regional versus systemic continuous 5-fluorodeoxyuridine chemotherapy in the treatment of colorectal liver metastases. *Ann Surg* 1987; 206: 685-93.
19. Cancer M-AGI: Reappraisal of hepatic infusion in the treatment of liver metases from colorectal cancer. *J Natl Cancer Inst* 1996; 88: 252-86.

III

Cost-effective strategies in tumor staging and imaging

Update Gastroenterology 2000.
Arnold R., Galmiche J.P., eds. John Libbey Eurotext, Paris © 2000, pp. 77-84.

Staging and imaging of esophageal and gastric carcinoma

Andreas Sendler, Hubert J. Stein, J. Rüdiger Siewert

Chirurgische Klinik und Poliklinik, Klinikum rechts der Isar der TU München, München, Germany

A tailored therapeutic approach requires exact pretherapeutic staging for selection of the adequate treatment modality [1]. After histologic confirmation and exact topographic localization of a malignant tumor, the determination of the depth of tumor infiltration into the organ wall (T category), the lymph node status (N category) and the presence or absence of distant metastases (M category) thus become essential. Especially in times with limited financial resources, the meticulous selection of patients for often time consuming and expensive therapies is of growing importance. In the following, we will discus cost-effective strategies in staging and imaging. It should be mentioned that the most cost-sparing approach is still the best diagnosis possible to select adequate treatment and/or to exclude incurable patients from incriminating or even useless therapies.

Esophageal carcinoma

Information on the localization of the tumor should be available before applying the TNM-staging. Tumors above or at the tracheal bifurcation and those tumors below have to be differentiated, as the localization has distinct impact on the possibility of resection. The limitation of esophageal resection is the tracheo-bronchial tree. Both organs are located very closely in the upper half, not leaving space for real radical resection, except in early tumor stages (T1/T2). For this reason bronchoscopy is mandatory in suprabifurcal carcinomas, since tumor invasion of the wall of the tracheo-bronchial tree can only be documented by this method. If the tumor has already infiltrated the tracheal wall, it is to be considered unresectable in a less advantaged stage than the infrabifurcal tumor [2].

T-category

Using video endoscopy and endoscopic ultrasound (EUS) the macroscopic tumor appearance and the infiltration of the wall can be precisely evaluated. The invasion of the wall is visualized with a high accuracy by the endoluminal ultrasound (EUS). In our own experience, the diagnostic accuracy of this method was 81% in T1, 77% in T2, 89% in T3 and 88% in T4 cases [3]. The overall accuracy of EUS in comparison to CT in esophageal cancer is shown in *Table I*. However, the use of EUS in esophageal cancer however is hampered by two problems:
- the possibility of overstaging a tumor. It is sometimes difficult to differentiate between cancer, inflamed surrounding soft tissue and fibrous changes. In a group of 167 cases, we found 17% cases over- or understaged, mainly in the T1 and T2 groups;
- in around 30% of esophageal carcinomas, tumorgrowth leads to a non-passable stenosis. However, two studies [3, 4] showed that in these cases a T3- or T4-stage was present in about 88% of patients, leading to a staging sensitivity of 85%, in T3 and 84% in T4 carcinoma.

N-category

The evaluation of the N-stages is more difficult, as EUS can only visualize lymph nodes in a close vicinity to the esophageal wall. In our own experience we found a sensitivity of 75% and a specificity of 70%. However, as shown in *table I*, EUS is still more sensitive when compared to CT scan, whereas sensitivity ranges between 51% and 74%.

Table I. Accuracy of EUS for local staging of esophageal cancer in comparison with CT (modified from [11]).

		Accuracy (%)	
Stage	n	EUS	CT
T1, T2	42	74	36
T3	95	93	74
T4	73	93	47
N0	55	64	73
N1	125	88	48

M-category

Esophageal cancer metastasizes early. The organs most frequently affected by distant metastases are the liver (32%), the lung (21%) and abdominal lymph nodes, particularly those of the celiac axis (6%). Distant metastases are detected using CT scan and percutaneous abdominal ultrasound (US). Spiral CT scan is currently the best method to detect metastases in these organs, as well as in the distant lymph nodes (M_{Lym}), *e.g.* in the celiac axis.

Percutaneous ultrasonography, plain chest X-rays and CT scanning are usually employed to assess distant metastases. Even with modern imaging technology small metastases (< 1 cm in diameter) are, however, often missed. Recent studies indicate that positron emission tomography detects many of these systemic tumor manifestations. In patients with adenocarcinoma of the distal esophagus, the shortcomings of standard imaging techniques in the detection of peritoneal carcinosis or small liver metastases can be overcome by diagnostic laparoscopy with laparoscopic ultrasound. In patients with squamous cell esophageal cancer the additional information obtained by diagnostic laparoscopy is marginal [5].

If neoadjuvant therapy is considered, the patient also needs to be evaluated for adequate liver, renal and bone marrow function. Since preoperative radiation or combined radiochemotherapy appears to increase postoperative morbidity after an esophagectomy, a thorough evaluation of the physiologic reserve and the general status is essential in these patients to make sure that they can withstand a potentially prolonged and complicated postoperative course. In our experience, a detailed risk analysis employing a dedicated organ function scoring system has proved helpful in selecting such patients [6].

Figure 1 and *2* display a diagnostic approach to squamous cell carcinoma and adenocarcinoma of the esophagus. This approach allows the identification of a group of patients with locally advanced tumors who may benefit from multimodal therapy [7, 8].

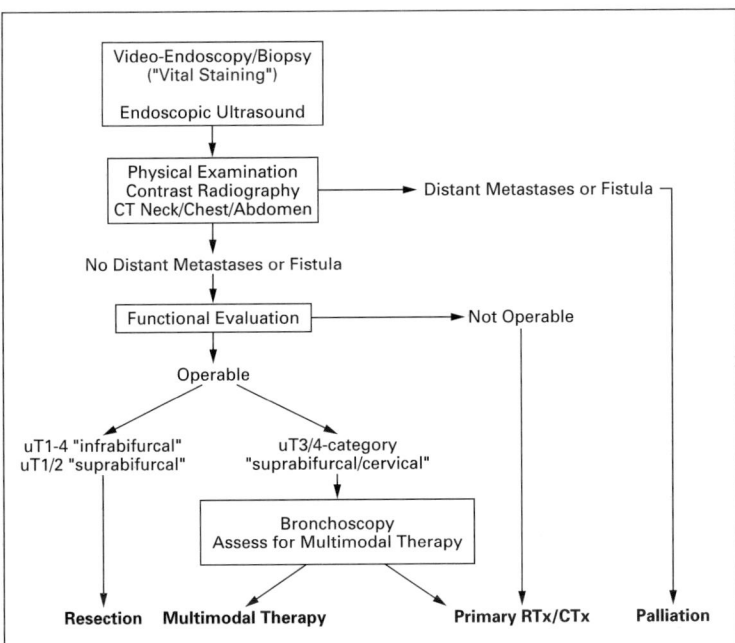

Figure 1. Diagnostic and individualised therapeutic approach to patients with squamous cell carcinoma of the esophagus.

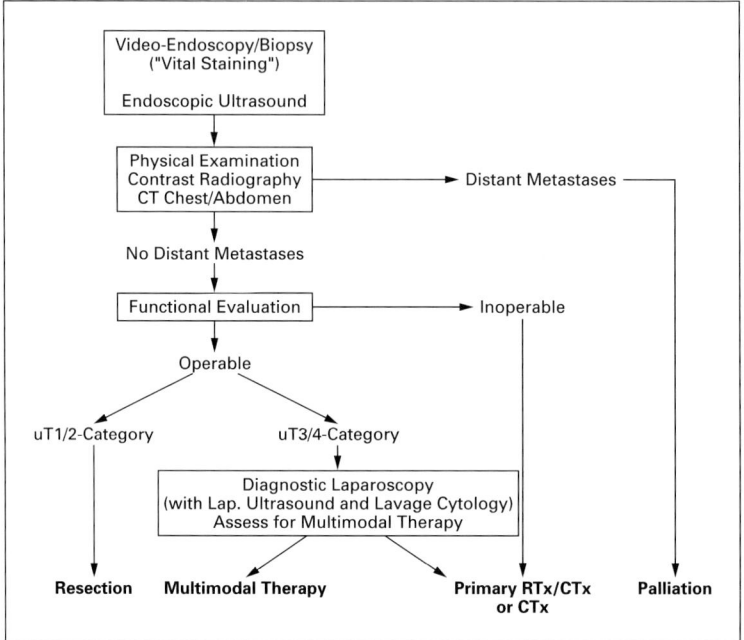

Figure 2. Diagnostic and individualised therapeutic approach to patients with adenocarcinoma of the esophagus.

Gastric carcinoma

T-category

Using endoscopy and biopsy, the location of the tumor and its macroscopic appearance should be clarified. Early gastric cancer and advanced gastric cancer (Borrmann classification) are classified differently according to the Japanese Gastric Cancer Association [9]. The localization of the tumor is crucial, as it determines different surgical strategies.

Carcinoma of the proximal gastric third can frequently not be differentiated from the true carcinoma of the cardia. In addition, these tumors must be distinguished from adenocarcinoma of the distal esophagus (the so-called Barrett's carcinoma). In our experience, these three tumor entities of the esophago-gastric junction (AEG) can be best discriminated based on the location of the tumor center [10]. The diagnosis of a Barrett's carcinoma (AEG type I) is usually easy, because the accompanying columnar type epithelium can be documented in 75 - 85% of patients. At least two thirds of the tumor mass must be located in the tubular esophagus to classify a tumor as Barrett's carcinoma. To classify a tumor as proximal gastric carcinoma (AEG type III), the tumor center must be aboral of the anatomic cardia. Tumors whose center is located within 2 cm oral or aboral of the anatomic cardia consequently represent the true carcinomas of the cardia (AEG type II). With regard to therapy, it is only necessary to definitely differentiate the Barrett's carcinoma from the other two entities. This is because a Barrett's carcinoma must be treated as esophageal cancer, while the therapeutic principles are similar for the true carcinoma of the cardia and tumors of the proximal gastric third. The different types of adenocarcinoma of the esophago-gastric junction (AEG type I-III) are displayed in *figure 3* [10]. For staging of adenocarcinoma of the esophagus, see above.

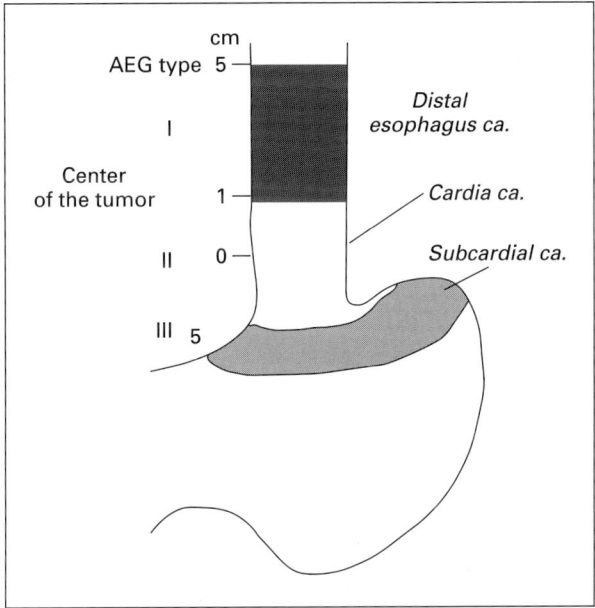

Figure 3. Definition of adenocarcinoma of the esophago-gastric junction (AEG type I-III).

Since the depth of infiltration is one of the most important prognostic factors also in gastric cancer, endoluminal ultrasound (EUS) is the first step for further diagnostic planning. The overall diagnostic accuracy of staging the T category using EUS is about 85% *(table II)* [11]. Problems still arise in the differentiation of T2 (subserosal invasion) from the T3 stage. This distinction is crucial, since it separates local from the locally advanced tumor growth. The use of EUS is sill hampered by the problem of over- or understaging. It is often difficult, especially in ulcerated gastric cancer, to differentiate between carcinoma, inflamed surrounding soft tissue or even fibrosis. Furthermore, EUS cannot detect micro-invasive cancer [12]. In this context, it has to be mentioned that the use of EUS is strongly dependent on the training and experience of the investigator. Further evaluation of the method must be carried out with respect to clinical consequences and its value in daily routine praxis. EUS is still far superior to CT for the determination of the overall T category. Lightdale [13] found a concordance of 92% between EUS and surgical pathology and only 42% concordance for CT scan.

There is no specific serum tumor marker for gastric cancer. However, carcinoembryonic antigen levels and CA 72-4 are frequently elevated in patients with extensive disease and may be used as a marker in monitoring the progress during treatment.

Table II. Accuracy of EUS locoregional staging in gastric cancer by stage (TNM 1992) [11].

Stage	n	Accuracy (%) EUS
T1	483	86
T2	301	64
T3	500	91
T4	143	80
N0	282	85
N1	311	71
N2	232	65

N-category

Using EUS, the diagnostic accuracy of determining the N-category according to the old TNM classification (up to 1998) in gastric cancer is reported to be 65%-87%. The diagnosis of lymph node metastases is problematic due to a low rate of detected lymph nodes and a high rate of false-positive findings. EUS can only visualize lymph nodes in close proximity to the gastric wall. As with other imaging methods, EUS can only detect enlarged lymph nodes. Nodes that are invaded but not enlarged cannot be detected. Furthermore it is not possible to count lymph nodes by EUS. Therefore it is recommended to stage the nodal status only as N positive (+) or negative. However, there is a distinct correlation between the T category and the number and localization of invaded lymph nodes. T3 tumors have a possibility of 88% positive lymph nodes. Overall, EUS is still more accurate than percutaneous ultrasound or CT for the evaluation of N stage.

Of particular interest is that the possibility of lymph node involvement and the prediction of the individual prognosis of gastric cancer can be predicted with the help of a validated and well established computer program [14].

M-category

Due to the embryonic rotation of the stomach, gastric cancer metastasizes not only into the lymph nodes of the greater and lesser omentum, but also into the lymph nodes around the celiac axis and the retroperitoneal space along the large abdominal vessels. The tumor itself can reach "per continuitatem" liver, pancreas, small and large bowel and sometimes the spleen. Seldom, in about 3% of the cases, the tumor metastasizes primarily to the bone marrow. In female patients, metastases at the ovary are a possible additional finding (Krukenberg tumors). The different subtypes of the Laurén classification have different patterns of metastasation. While the intestinal type metastasizes preferentially to the liver and lymph nodes, the diffuse type spreads into the peritoneum [15]. Taking these routes of tumor spread into account, CT-examination of the whole abdominal cavity is necessary. However, a very crucial region for distant spread of gastric cancer, the peritoneum, can only be visualized using CT scanning when ascites is present.

Conventional ultrasonography (US), Spiral CT scanning and MRI are the choice methods for detecting liver metastases. Small metastases (< 1 cm in diameter) pose a serious problem because they evade established diagnostic methods, and are the predominantly size of metastases which are found. The sensitivity of US and CT for detecting the presence or absence of metastatic disease in the liver is about 85% [16]. However, for the identification of individual lesions, the sensitivity of these techniques is considerably lower. About one in three lesions is missed, usually lesions under 1 cm in diameter.

The described pitfalls in staging can be overcome by surgical laparoscopy. Peritoneal spread of a tumor is easily visualized and confirmed by a video-guided biopsy. In an own study, peritoneal carcinomatosis was found in 23% of 111 patients during laparoscopy, which was undetected after conventional staging. Intra-laparoscopic ultrasound furthermore even makes possible the detection of small (< 1 cm) liver metastases [17]. In addition, laparoscopy provides the possibility of obtaining an abdominal lavage to detect so-called free tumor cells in the abdominal cavity. With the use of immunohistochemical staining, the cytological evaluation of lavage fluid provides even more valuable information [18].

The staging is completed with a bone scintigram (for T3/T4 tumors) and a chest X-ray. *Figure 4* displays a diagnostic approach to gastric cancer based on preoperative staging. This approach allows the identification of a group of patients with locally advanced gastric carcinoma who may benefit from preoperative chemotherapy [19].

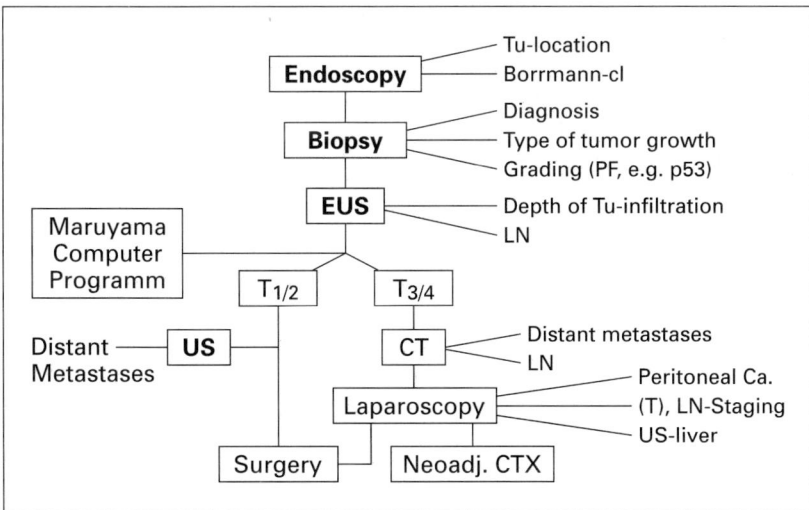

Figure 4. Flow chart illustrating the diagnostic evaluation for patients with gastric cancer in oncologic centers prepared to provide multimodal treatment (PF: prognostic factors, CTX: chemotherapy)

References

1. Siewert JR, Sendler A, Dittler HJ, Fink U, Höfler H. Staging gastrointestinal cancer as a precondition for multimodal treatment. *World J Surg* 1995; 19: 168-77.
2. Siewert JR, Dittler HJ. Esophageal carcinoma: impact of staging on treatment. *Endoscopy* 1993; 25: 28-32.
3. Dittler HJ, Siewert JR. Role of endoscopic ultrasonography in esophageal carcinoma. *Endoscopy* 1993; 25: 156-61.
4. Rösch T, Lorenz R, Zenker K, von Wichert A, Dancygier H, Hofler H et al. Local staging and assessment of resectability in carcinoma of the esophagus, stomach, and duodenum by endoscopic ultrasonography. *Gastrointest Endosc* 1992; 38: 460-7.
5. Stein HJ, Kraemer SJ, Feussner H, Fink U, Siewert JR. Clinical Value of Diagnostic Laparoscopy With Laparoscopic Ultrasound in Patients With Cancer of the Esophagus or Cardia. *J Gastrointest Surg* 1997; 1: 167-73.
6. Bartels H, Stein HJ, Siewert JR. Risk analysis in esophageal surgery. *Recent Results Cancer Res* 2000; 155: 89-96.
7. Siewert JR, Stein HJ, Sendler A, Fink U. Surgical resection for cancer of the cardia. *Semin Surg Oncol* 1999; 17: 125-31.
8. Siewert JR, Stein HJ, Sendler A. Chirurgische Relevanz bildgebender Diagnostik bei Tumoren des Gastrointestinaltrakts - Entscheidungswege beim Esophagus- Magen-, Colon- und Rectumkarzinom. *Chirurg* 1997; 68: 317-24.
9. Japanese Research Society for Gastric Cancer. The general rules for the gastric cancer study in surgery and pathology I: Clinical classification. *Jpn J Surg* 1981; 11: 127-39.
10. Siewert JR, Stein HJ. Classification of adenocarcinoma of the esophagogastric junction. *Br J Surg* 1998; 85: 1457-9.
11. Rösch Th. Endosonographic staging of gastric cancer: a review of literature results. *Gastrointest Clin North Am* 1995; 3: 549-57.
12. Pollack BJ, Chak A, Sivak MV, Jr. Endoscopic ultrasonography. *Semin Oncol* 1996; 23: 336-46.
13. Lightdale CJ. Endoscopic ultrasonography in the diagnosis, staging and follow-up of esophageal and gastric cancer. *Endoscopy* 1992; 24 Suppl 1: 297-303.
14. Maruyama K, Gunven P, Okabayashi K, Sasako M, Kinoshita T. Lymph node metastases of gastric cancer. General pattern in 1931 patients. *Ann Surg* 1989; 210: 596-602.
15. Weiss M, Eder M, Bassermann R. Charakterisierung verschiedener Magenkarzinomtypen mit unterschiedlicher Metastasierung in Leber, Peritoneum und Knochen. *Pathology* 1993; 14: 260-4.
16. Saini S. Imaging of the hepatobiliary tract. *N Engl J Med* 1997; 336: 1889-94.
17. Feussner H, Kraemer SJM, Siewert JR. Staging-Laparoskopie. *Chirurg* 1997; 68: 201-9.
18. Nekarda H, Gess C, Stark M, Mueller JD, Fink U, Schenck U et al. Immunocytochemically detected free peritoneal tumour cells (FPTC) are a strong prognostic factor in gastric carcinoma. *Br J Cancer* 1999; 79: 611-9.
19. Sendler A, Dittler HJ, Feussner H, Nekarda H, Bollschweiler E, Fink U et al. Preoperative staging of gastric cancer as precondition for multimodal treatment. *World J Surg* 1995; 19: 501-8.

Staging and imaging of pancreatic cancer

Kaspar Z'graggen, Bruno M. Schmied, Helmut Friess, Markus W. Büchler

*Department of Visceral and Transplantation Surgery, Inselspital,
University of Bern, Switzerland*

Surgery plays a key role in the treatment of patients with pancreatic cancer and it is at present the only modality with a chance for long-term survival. Curative surgery can be performed in 40-70% of patients referred to institutions specialized in pancreatic surgery. For patients presenting with pancreatic cancer, staging of the disease is essential. Different factors, such as the risk profile of the patient, the availability of imaging modalities, the case load of pancreatic diseases and the level of endoscopic and surgical expertise can impact on the treatment strategy for such patients and determine cost effectiveness.

Preoperative staging should ideally distinguish resectable from unresectable disease and identify patients that are best managed by palliative non-surgical treatment. Metastatic and locally invasive pancreatic cancer is usually not amenable to resection [1, 2]. Therefore the detection of tumor spread into distant organs or locally into vascular structures is an integral part of staging procedures. Resectability is often determined during explorative laparotomy but recent advances in radiological and endoscopic techniques and diagnostic laparoscopy improved assessment of tumor extension prior to laparotomy. This article discusses the rationale of different preoperative staging strategies for patients with pancreatic cancer and their value for a cost effective approach.

Case load and cost effectiveness

Quality and efficiency in the treatment of pancreatic cancer depend on the volume of patients treated. Recent publications analyzed the relation between the patient volume, outcome and cost effectiveness [3, 4]. A correlation between the number of pancreatic resections, morbidity and in-hospital mortality has repeatedly been shown and a recent publication also demonstrated that high volume centers have lower cost [5-7]. Although these data confirm the volume-outcome relationship in other areas of interest including colorectal and liver surgery and urology [6, 8], hospital experience is particularly important with pancreaticoduodenectomy. There is good evidence that patients considering this procedure should be given the option of care at a high-volume referral center [5, 9]. However, the patient with suspected pancreatic cancer usually presents to a physician or institution that does not focus on hepato-biliary and pancreatic diseases and at present more than half of these patients are treated at low volume institutions performing two or less pancreatoduodenectomies per year [10].

Initial approach to a patient with suspected pancreatic cancer

Painless jaundice is the typical presentation of a patient with cancer of the pancreatic head. Ultrasonography (US) is often used as the first imaging modality; it is relatively inexpensive but has considerable observer variability as its main disadvantage. US has the ability to detect small liver metastases of five millimeters or less, but in a patient with suspected pancreatic cancer, US is more important to diagnose or exclude gallstone disease and does not provide all staging information necessary to determine the patients treatment strategy.

The standard imaging procedure for pancreatic cancer is at present contrast enhanced abdominal computed tomography (CT) with an early arterial phase and it usually determines size and location of the tumor, the presence of liver metastases and occasionally ascites and peritoneal metastases. Conventional anteroposterior and lateral chest radiography is generally sufficient to detect pulmonary metastases. However, magnetic resonance tomography (MR), if available in high quality, has the added advantage of MR cholangio-pancreatography (MRCP) and MR angiography [11]. While MR may be the standard first line imaging procedure in the future, abdominal CT scan is less expensive and certainly more readily available at present. CT and MR detect more than 80% of distant metastasis from pancreatic cancer corresponding to UICC stage IVb. In the following, different staging exams are discussed in terms of accuracy to distinguish patients with resectable pancreatic cancer (UICC stages I-III) from patients with unresectable disease, either because of local tumor extension leading to irresectablility or because of previously unknown metastases to the liver or peritoneal cavity.

Endoscopic ultrasound

Endoscopic ultrasound (EUS) is a promising new staging technique that may detect small tumors of the pancreatic head and sometimes allows their exact localization and extension [12]. Vascular involvement (T4) can be assessed by color Doppler US with high accuracy (91%) [13] and infiltration of duodenum and peripancreatic tissue can be detected in pancreatic cancer [14]. Its use is currently limited to specialized institutions and the quality of EUS is even more observer-dependent than in US. The impact of EUS findings on treatment strategy in pancreatic cancer is currently limited. It does not improve detection of metastases and its accuracy to distinguish vascular infiltration by the tumor from inflammatory peritumorous reaction is too low. In selected patients EUS may confirm extensive vascular infiltration in the superior mesenteric and portal vein. Furthermore, most specialized institutions do not recommend percutaneous fine needle aspiration, because of the potential of tumor seeding, but EUS guided fine needle aspiration leaves the needle tract in the future pancreatoduodenectomy specimen and may therefore be performed. Lymph node size is not a reliable indicator for the presence of metastasis, and differentiation between reactive and malignant lymph nodes is notoriously difficult and the presence of lymph node metastasis does not exclude patients from potentially curative surgery [15].

Computed tomography scan

We discussed above that abdominal CT scan is an effective imaging exam in a patient with suspected pancreatic cancer and standardization of spiral abdominal CT improved tumor staging of pancreatic cancer [16]. Its accuracy to diagnose pancreatic cancer is more than 90% [17] because benign solid pancreatic tumors are rare. The distinction between malignancy and an inflammatory mass of the pancreatic head in a patient with chronic pancreatitis may be difficult [18].

The ability of abdominal CT scan to determine resectability and unresectability of pancreatic cancer is currently an unresolved issue. In a recent study, it allowed to predict tumor resectability in 72% and its sensitivity and specificity for unresectability was 78% and 76%, respectively [19, 20]. Although its predictive value for vascular infiltration was 88% in a recent publication [20], the radiological assessment of local tumor extension is difficult, since the degree of vascular encasement and institutional resectability rates are variable [21-23]. A patient with a potentially resectable pancreatic tumor should undergo surgical exploration, and unresectability should currently be determined by the surgeon's assessment of the staging exams and intraoperatively. Tumors in the head of the pancreas can also originate within the ampullary tissue (papilla, distal common bile duct, duodenum) and these cancers behave differently in terms of tumor biology and have a more favorable outcome and a higher resection rate. The prognostic value of CT in these patients is therefore more limited.

Endoscopic retrograde cholangiopancreatography (ERCP)

Clinically jaundiced patients with pancreatic malignancy often undergo ERCP that allows definition of biliary pathology and alterations of the main pancreatic duct and its side branches with an accuracy of 95% [24]. ERCP is the gold standard in the detection of subtle pancreatic and biliary abnormalities such as *in situ* tumors and T1 tumors but its value for preoperative tumor staging is low [14]. The possibility to biopsy ductal pathology, collect samples for cytologic analysis and place stents or nasobiliary drains to relief obstructive jaundice are often used in patients with cancer of the head of the pancreas. ERCP and endoscopic placing of biliary stents in patients with potentially resectable tumors are probably not cost-effective although the preoperative drainage of the obstructed common bile duct is still debated. In patients with tumors of the body and tail of the pancreas, ERCP does not impact on staging or treatment strategy.

Endoscopic stent placing as definitive treatment in patients with stage IV pancreatic cancer is recommended by many authors ; it has the advantage of a usually short hospital stay, and avoids operation. However, the frequently necessary exchange of plastic stents and the morbidity and cost of these procedures and associated hospital stays have to be compared to more recent data of bypass surgery that demonstrate very low mortality with acceptable morbidity and a short hospital stay [25-27].

Magnetic resonance imaging and angiography

Magnetic resonance imaging (MR) including MR cholangiopancreatography and MR-angiography [11] has the potential to replace CT scan in combination with diagnostic ERCP as the primary imaging modality for staging of pancreatic cancer. In some patients it allows the detection of tumors smaller than 1 cm in diameter [28]. However, since many pancreatic tumors are not diagnosed with screening exams, the sensitivity for small non-symptomatic tumors is not its main advantage. The ability of MR to define tumor extension in relation to vascular structures non-invasively makes MR attractive for preoperative assessment. The reduction of cost and time of examination will in the future facilitate its routine application. MR-angiography also replaced conventional angiography, a technique that was regularly used in patients with pancreatic cancer but that has lost its importance in preoperative staging.

Diagnostic laparoscopy

All non-invasive staging examinations have a false negative rate of 10-30% for small liver and/or peritoneal metastases [29, 30]. Diagnostic laparoscopy has been advocated to avoid unnecessary laparotomy and/or to prove the malignant nature of hepatobiliary and pancreatic tumors by biopsy. Its routine use has been advocated for patients with pancreatic cancer, and in particular for patients with tumors of the pancreatic body and tail. These cancers usually present in advanced stages, are rarely resectable, and peritoneal metastases can often be found intraoperatively. Laparoscopy can improve tumor staging but its value for the determination of resectability is questioned. In pancreatic cancer, detection of metastatic lesions by laparoscopy has been reported in 10% to 35% [30-32]. The value of concurrent peritoneal lavage cytology and immunohistochemical examination that approximately doubles the detection of minimal peritoneal tumor spread has not been defined conclusively. We recommend diagnostic laparoscopy only as a selective staging procedure in patients with locally advanced non-metastatic cancer because in more than 75% of our pancreatic cancer patients, laparoscopy did not change course of treatment and allowed detection of abdominal metastases in only 10% [31]. The routine use of diagnostic laparoscopy is therefore not cost effective.

Discussion

The preoperative assessment of patients with pancreatic cancer includes tumor staging and registration of operative risks, particularly preexisting cardiopulmonary disease. This allows to determine a treatment strategy, in particular whether to attempt curative or palliative treatment. Potentially curative surgery is defined by a radical resection (R0) of the primary tumor and includes lymphadenectomy. Morbidity and mortality rates of pancreatic resections decreased to less than five percent in many specialized centers and more radical resections to improve long-term survival can be performed [33-35]. While this approach significantly improved survival of patients with hepatobiliary cancer [36], prospective randomized studies on radical surgery in pancreatic cancer have not conclusively determined the extent needed [37, 38], and further studies are planned. Preoperative staging primarily includes radiological imaging, but molecular techniques of tumor-associated antigens, monoclonal antibodies, cytokines, genetic markers and the detection of minimal cancer spread in blood, bone marrow and the peritoneal cavity are currently under investigation and may in the future improve staging.

Cost-effectiveness has not been extensively studied for staging strategies in pancreatic cancer but there is evidence in pancreatic surgery and for other complex surgical procedures that the volume of patients treated is a major determinant of outcome. Volume or caseload affect morbidity, mortality, hospital stay and long-term survival and directly relate to cost [25]. If pancreatic cancer is suspected, the cost-effective strategy at present is to perform an abdominal CT scan, or a high quality MRI including MRCP if painless jaundice is present.

New diagnostic tools have improved preoperative staging and allow a more accurate definition of local tumor extension, and further technical developments can be expected. However, available tools, such as EUS, do not always impact on treatment strategy. There are many valid indications for EUS in pancreatic diseases such as the localization of endocrine tumors and assessment of cystic pancreatic tumors, but in patients with pancreatic cancer routine application is certainly not within the concept of cost-effectiveness.

The key information for the surgeon collected by staging studies, pertains to the presence of metastases and definitive signs of unresectability, such as a complex infiltration of vascular structures [39]. Resectability is still defined intraoperatively and resection in a curative attempt is often possible despite a close relation of the tumor to vital vessels. Advances in surgical technique such as the safe resection and reanastomosis of portal structures, have extended the spectrum of surgical indications towards more advanced tumors and lead to a considerable reduction of both, morbidity and mortality [33]. Long-term survival can be achieved in more than 20% of patients undergoing radical resection for pancreatic cancer [40, 41]. In patients with nonresectable pancreatic cancer and distant metastases, endoscopic stent placing can be recommended. However, the cost effectiveness of this approach may have to be controlled when specialized referral centers are available for pancreatic cancer patients that demonstrate low morbidity and mortality rates of 1% or less for surgical bypass procedures [42].

Summary and algorithm of cost-effective staging

At present the cost-effective staging approach in patients with suspected pancreatic cancer is to perform an abdominal ultrasound that allows the diagnosis of a biliary pathology and is sensitive for the detection of liver metastasis *(figure 1)*. Helical CT scan is currently

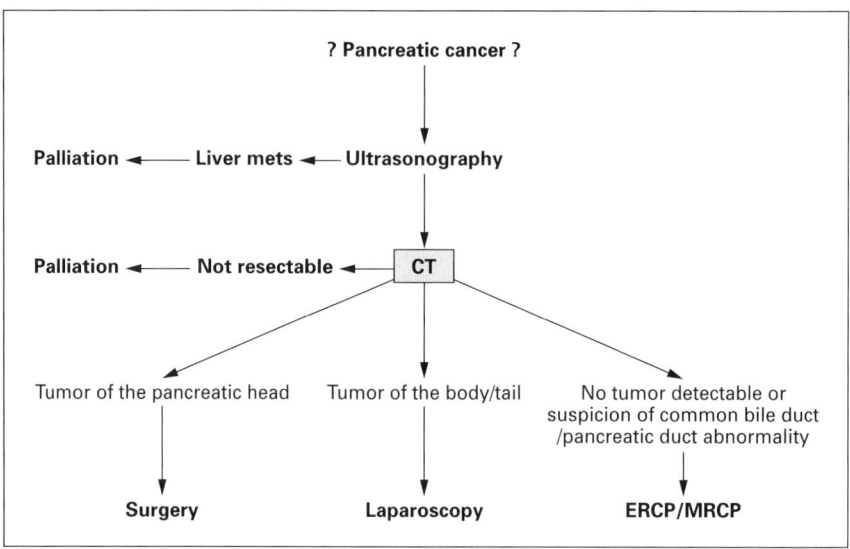

Figure 1. Algorithm of cost-effective pancreatic cancer staging.

the staging examination that provides the most pertinent information to the treatment of pancreatic cancer patients and is widely available. The detected pathology and its localization usually allow to decide whether patients with suspected pancreatic cancer need explorative surgery, laparoscopy or further staging examinations such as ERCP or MRCP. EUS, a relatively new staging examination, is important for mostly benign pancreatic diseases and cystic tumors, but its routine use in pancreatic cancer is currently not cost-effective. In the future, EUS and MRI may further improve staging and in particular determine complex infiltration into vascular structures.

References

1. Fuhrman GM, Leach SD, Staley CA, Cusack JC, Charnsangavej C, Cleary KR, El-Naggar AK, Fenoglio CJ, Lee JE, Evans DB. Rationale for en bloc vein resection in the treatment of pancreatic adenocarcinoma adherent to the superior mesenteric-portal vein confluence. Pancreatic Tumor Study Group. *Ann Surg* 1996; 223: 154-62.
2. Hemmingsson A, Jacobson G, Lindgren PG, Lonnerholm T, Lorelius LE, Nordgren CE. Radiologic assessment of resectability of carcinoma of the head of the pancreas. *Acta Radiol [Diagn]* 1982; 23: 127-30.
3. Richter JM, Barry MJ. Decision analysis for the practicing gastroenterologist. 2. Insights into the efficacy of diagnostic strategies using decision analysis. *Am J Gastroenterol* 1985; 80: 493-7.
4. Elixhauser A, Halpern MT. Economic evaluations of gastric and pancreatic cancer. *Hepatogastroenterology* 1999; 46: 1206-13.
5. Begg CB, Cramer LD, Hoskins WJ, Brennan MF. Impact of hospital volume on operative mortality for major cancer surgery [see comments]. *Jama* 1998; 280: 1747-51.
6. Choti MA, Bowman HM, Pitt HA, Sosa JA, Sitzmann JV, Cameron JL, Gordon TA. Should hepatic resections be performed at high-volume referral centers? *J Gastrointest Surg* 1998; 2: 11-20.

7. Birkmeyer JD, Finlayson SR, Tosteson AN, Sharp SM, Warshaw AL, Fisher ES. Effect of hospital volume on in-hospital mortality with pancreaticoduodenectomy [see comments]. *Surgery* 1999; 125: 250-6.
8. Ellison LM, Heaney JA, Birkmeyer JD. The effect of hospital volume on mortality and resource use after radical prostatectomy. *J Urol* 2000; 163: 867-9.
9. Kingsnorth AN. Major HPB procedures must be undertaken in high volume quaternary centres? *HPB Surg* 2000; 11: 359-61.
10. Gordon TA, Bowman HM, Tielsch JM, Bass EB, Burleyson GP, Cameron JL. Statewide regionalization of pancreaticoduodenectomy and its effect on in-hospital mortality. *Ann Surg* 1998; 228: 71-8.
11. Trede M, Rumstadt B, Wendl K, Gaa J, Tesdal K, Lehmann KJ, Meier-Willersen HJ, Pescatore P, Schmoll J. Ultrafast magnetic resonance imaging improves the staging of pancreatic tumors. *Ann Surg* 1997; 226: 393-405; discussion 405-7.
12. Brugge WR, Van Dam J. Pancreatic and biliary endoscopy. *N Engl J Med* 1999; 341: 1808-16.
13. Smits NJ, Reeders JW. Imaging and staging of biliopancreatic malignancy: role of ultrasound. *Ann Oncol* 1999; 10: 20-4.
14. Tio TL, Wijers OB, Sars PR, Tytgat GN. Preoperative TNM classification of proximal extrahepatic bile duct carcinoma by endosonography. *Semin Liver Dis* 1990; 10: 114-20.
15. Smits NJ, Reeders JW. Current applicability of duplex Doppler ultrasonography in pancreatic head and biliary malignancies. *Baillieres Clin Gastroenterol* 1995; 9: 153-72.
16. Bluemke DA, Fishman EK. CT and MR evaluation of pancreatic cancer. *Surg Oncol Clin N Am* 1998; 7: 103-24.
17. Baer H, Wagner M, Büchler M. Onkologische Standardchirurgie des Pankreaskarzinoms. *Chir Gastroenterol* 1998; 14: 42-8.
18. Beger HG, Buchler M. Duodenum-preserving resection of the head of the pancreas in chronic pancreatitis with inflammatory mass in the head. *World J Surg* 1990; 14: 83-7.
19. Saldinger PF, Reilly M, Reynolds K, Raptopoulos V, Chuttani R, Steer ML, Matthews JB. Is CT angiography sufficient for prediction of resectability of periampullary neoplasms? *J Gastrointest Surg* 2000; 4: 233-7; discussion 238-9.
20. Phoa SS, Reeders JW, Rauws EA, De Wit L, Gouma DJ, Lameris JS. Spiral computed tomography for preoperative staging of potentially resectable carcinoma of the pancreatic head. *Br J Surg* 1999: 86: 789-94.
21. Warshaw AL, Gu ZY, Wittenberg J, Waltman AC. Preoperative staging and assessment of resectability of pancreatic cancer. *Arch Surg* 1990; 125: 230-3.
22. Gmeinwieser J, Feuerbach S, Hohenberger W, Albrich H, Strotzer M, Hofstadter F, Geissler A. Spiral-CT in diagnosis of vascular involvement in pancreatic cancer. *Hepatogastroenterology* 1995; 42: 418-22.
23. Hough TJ, Raptopoulos V, Siewert B, Matthews JB. Teardrop superior mesenteric vein: CT sign for unresectable carcinoma of the pancreas. *AJR Am J Roentgenol* 1999; 173: 1509-12.
24. Spinelli P, Schiavo M, Schicchi AA. [Endoscopy in the diagnosis and staging of pancreatic cancer]. *Tumori* 1999; 85: S14-8.
25. Sosa JA, Bowman HM, Gordon TA, Bass EB, Yeo CJ, Lillemoe KD, Pitt HA, Tielsch JM, Cameron JL. Importance of hospital volume in the overall management of pancreatic cancer. *Ann Surg* 1998; 228: 429-38.
26. Gouma DJ, van Dijkum EJ, van Geenen RC, van Gulik TM, Obertop H. Are there indications for palliative resection in pancreatic cancer? *World J Surg* 1999; 23: 954-9.
27. Gouma DJ, van Geenen R, van Gulik T, de Wit LT, Obertop H. Surgical palliative treatment in bilio-pancreatic malignancy. *Ann Oncol* 1999; 10: 269-72.
28. Irie H, Honda H, Kaneko K, Kuroiwa T, Yoshimitsu K, Masuda K. Comparison of helical CT and MR imaging in detecting and staging small pancreatic adenocarcinoma. *Abdom Imaging* 1997; 22: 429-33.

29. Warshaw AL, Tepper JE, Shipley WU. Laparoscopy in the staging and planning of therapy for pancreatic cancer. *Am J Surg* 1986; 151: 76-80.
30. Fernandez-del Castillo C, Rattner DW, Warshaw AL. Further experience with laparoscopy and peritoneal cytology in the staging of pancreatic cancer. *Br J Surg* 1995; 82: 1127-9.
31. Friess H, Kleeff J, Silva JC, Sadowski C, Baer HU, Buchler MW. The role of diagnostic laparoscopy in pancreatic and periampullary malignancies. *J Am Coll Surg* 1998; 186: 675-82.
32. Makary MA, Warshaw AL, Centeno BA, Willet CG, Rattner DW, Fernandez-del Castillo C. Implications of peritoneal cytology for pancreatic cancer management. *Arch Surg* 1998; 133: 361-5.
33. Büchler M, Friess H, Wagner M. Pancreatic fistula after pancreatic head resection. *Br J Surg* 2000: in press.
34. Conlon KC, Klimstra DS, Brennan MF. Long-term survival after curative resection for pancreatic ductal adenocarcinoma. Clinicopathologic analysis of 5-year survivors. *Ann Surg* 1996; 223: 273-9.
35. Yeo CJ, Abrams RA, Grochow LB, Sohn TA, Ord SE, Hruban RH, Zahurak ML, Dooley WC, Coleman J, Sauter PK, Pitt HA, Lillemoe KD, Cameron JL. Pancreaticoduodenectomy for pancreatic adenocarcinoma: postoperative adjuvant chemoradiation improves survival. A prospective, single-institution experience. *Ann Surg* 1997; 225: 621-33; discussion 633-6.
36. Bartlett DL, Fong Y, Fortner JG, Brennan MF, Blumgart LH. Long-term results after resection for gallbladder cancer. Implications for staging and management. *Ann Surg* 1996; 224: 639-46.
37. Pedrazzoli S, DiCarlo V, Dionigi R, Mosca F, Pederzoli P, Pasquali C, Kloppel G, Dhaene K, Michelassi F. Standard versus extended lymphadenectomy associated with pancreatoduodenectomy in the surgical treatment of adenocarcinoma of the head of the pancreas: a multicenter, prospective, randomized study. Lymphadenectomy Study Group. *Ann Surg* 1998; 228: 508-17.
38. Yeo CJ, Cameron JL, Sohn TA, Coleman J, Sauter PK, Hruban RH, Pitt HA, Lillemoe KD. Pancreaticoduodenectomy with or without extended retroperitoneal lymphadenectomy for periampullary adenocarcinoma: comparison of morbidity and mortality and short-term outcome. *Ann Surg* 1999; 229: 613-22; discussion 622-4.
39. McCarthy MJ, Evans J, Sagar G, Neoptolemos JP. Prediction of resectability of pancreatic malignancy by computed tomography. *Br J Surg* 1998; 85: 320-5.
40. Bathe OF, Levi D, Caldera H, Franceschi D, Raez L, Patel A, Raub WA, Jr., Benedetto P, Reddy R, Hutson D, Sleeman D, Livingstone AS, Levi JU. Radical resection of periampullary tumors in the elderly: evaluation of long-term results. *World J Surg* 2000; 24: 353-8.
41. Trede M, Schwall G, Saeger HD. Survival after pancreatoduodenectomy. 118 consecutive resections without an operative mortality. *Ann Surg* 1990; 211: 447-58.
42. Van Wagensveld BA, Coene PP, van Gulik TM, Rauws EA, Obertop H, Gouma DJ. Outcome of palliative biliary and gastric bypass surgery for pancreatic head carcinoma in 126 patients [see comments]. *Br J Surg* 1997; 84: 1402-6.

Imaging modalities for diagnosis and staging of HCC

Ultrasound

The detection rate of HCC with ultrasound (US) is related to the size, location and echostructure of the lesion as well as the experience of the radiologist and the US technology employed. US has limited sensitivity for detecting HCC and limited specificity for the diagnosis of HCC in patients with cirrhosis because of significant overlap in the ultrasonographic appearance of benign nodules with small HCCs. However progress in US technology has improved detectability for small HCCs (measuring less than 2 cm in diameter) with a reported detection rate ranging from 46% to 95% [21, 22]. In the same studies, the detection rate of HCC measuring between 2 and 3 cm ranges from 82% to 93%. Tumor location can also influence the detection rate of HCCs. It has been demonstrated that the detection rate for tumors located in the anterior segments of the right lobe is about 10% higher than rates observed for the detection of tumors in the posterior segments of the right lobe [23]. In addition, detection and characterisation of lesions in posterior segments are not always precise enough to determine surgical strategies. The radiologist expertise is a crucial factor for an accurate assessment of liver lesions [24]. The detection rate of HCCs increased from 80% to 92% in the same group of patients when a more experienced examiner performed the examination [25].

The influence of tumor echogenicity on detectability has been well established. The presence of well defined margins or a perilesional halo, an hypoechoic pattern of the lesions are associated with a high rate of detection [26]. Conversely, infiltrative HCCs with iso or hyperechoic patterns, without peripheral halo, are more difficult to detect with reported sensitivities as low as 59% to 69% [26-28]. Indirect signs of the presence of tumor, such as vessel compression or protrusion of the liver capsule, may be useful when tumor echostructure is not different from the surrounding liver. However some diffuse HCCs are very difficult to identify, since the diffuse parenchymal inhomogeneity can be misinterpreted as being due to cirrhosis.

A frequent complication of HCC is vascular invasion by the neoplasm. Invasion of portal vessels occurred in up to 65% while invasion of the hepatic veins occurred in up to 30% of HCCs [29]. Vascular invasion can be used to detect the presence of HCCs not previously identified [30]. Doppler studies of hepatic vessels, which can be enhanced with contrast media, can be of help for differentiating between neoplastic and non-neoplastic thrombi: the presence of blood flow signals in the thrombi is highly suggestive of malignancy [31]. In addition, doppler studies can improve the characterisation of liver mass: many studies have shown that the specificity of this technique to differentiate malignant from benign liver tumors is quite high, up to 95% [32-34]. Indeed, unlike normal liver and precancerous primary liver lesions such as dysplastic nodules which are vascularized predominantly through portal circulation, HCCs are mostly supplied by arterial flow. The detection of arterial flow signals with colour-power doppler both around and inside a liver mass is highly suggestive of HCC [32, 33]. However, in either large or necrotic or small HCCs, a high rate of false negative diagnoses with Doppler studies can be explained by poor vascularization of the tumor.

Multifocal tumors are frequently observed in patients with HCC. Minute nodules located in the same segment or in an adjacent segment are considered daughter nodules. Multiple nodules located in both lobes are considered parts of a single multicentric tumor if none of them is large enough to be considered as the dominant mass. The remainder are considered intrahepatic metastases [35]. Most imaging modalities tend to underestimate the number of malignant lesions [36]. This point has been clearly demonstrated in the setting of liver transplantation by comparing pathological findings in liver explants to pretransplant imaging findings. It has been shown that US has very poor sensitivity, 45%, and very high specificity, 98%, for the detection of malignant tumors in a prospective study on 200 liver transplanted patients [37].

Computed tomography of the liver

The ability of computed tomography (CT) to depict liver tumors has increased during the past decade because of technologic advances and increased understanding of how to optimise CT techniques and contrast material administration. However, conventional contrast material-enhanced CT has been reported to depict only 50% to 80% of malignant liver lesions [38-40]. The development of helical CT scanner has provided the ability to scan the entire liver in a 20- to 30- second interval. Helical CT has rapidly become the standard in CT examination of the liver. One of the advantages of helical CT is a marked reduction in acquisition time, which allows the liver to be scanned twice during a short period of time. Therefore helical CT allows the separate imaging of the hepatic arterial phase and the portal venous phase. Because the liver receives 75% to 80% of its blood flow from the portal vein, imaging the liver during the hepatic arterial phase results in little enhancement of liver parenchyma. Hypervascular tumors such as HCC which receive almost all of their blood flow from the hepatic artery, receive only contrast-enhanced flow from the hepatic artery without dilution from the unenhanced portal vein during the hepatic arterial phase. Therefore they appear as enhanced masses which contrast with a minimally enhanced liver parenchyma for about 20 to 30 seconds *(figure 1)*. The hepatic capsule contour may be deformed by HCC *(figure 2)*. Imaging patients with HCC during the hepatic arterial phase will optimise tumor detection. Moreover, the coexistence of cirrhosis and altered portal venous blood flow on patients with HCC is an important reason why hepatic arterial phase imaging depicts more lesions than portal venous phase imaging. Portal venous blood flow is the predominant source of blood flow and contrast material delivery to the liver during the portal venous phase [41]. Therefore, portal venous phase imaging could be adversely affected by the decreased or hepatofugal flow in cirrhotic patient [42]. Currently, bi- or tri-phasic helical CT achieves a markedly higher detection rate for HCC (89% to 92%) than those obtained with conventional CT, especially for the detection of HCC smaller than 2 cm in size [16, 42-44]. However, helical CT may overestimate tumor staging. Indeed, it has been found that HCC is first enhanced following contrast injection. In a second time, the contrast agent enters the draining portal venules, which are seen as a halo around the mass. In other word, late phases CT images give an erroneously exaggerated size of tumor [45].

The use of lipiodol computed tomography, which is based on hepatic CT scan 2 weeks after intrahepatic arterial injection of lipiodol, has been reported to be highly sensitive for the detection of HCC [46, 47]. However, these reports are based on histological data obtained from resected specimens or needle biopsy rather than an evaluation of the whole

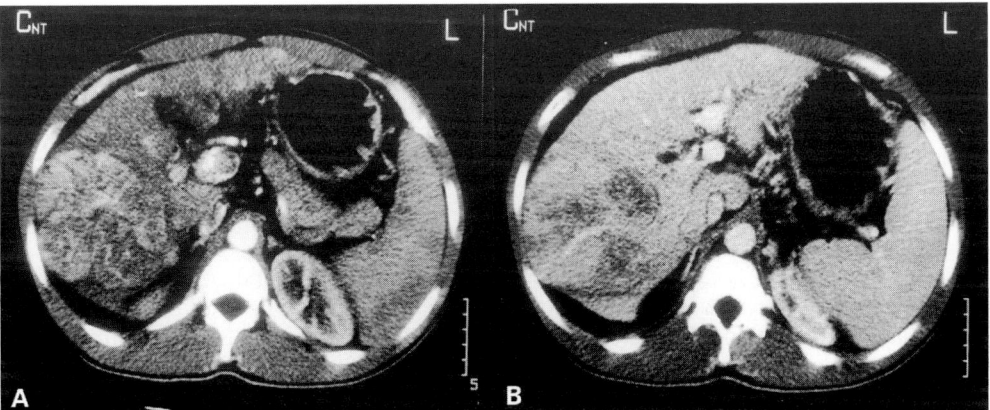

Figure 1. 65-year-old man with poorly differenciated hepatocellular carcinoma and cirrhosis documented after liver biopsy. (A) CT scan after injection of contrast material during arterial phase shows hyperdense mass. (B) CT scan after injection of contrast material during late phase shows heterogenous and hypodense mass of the right liver.

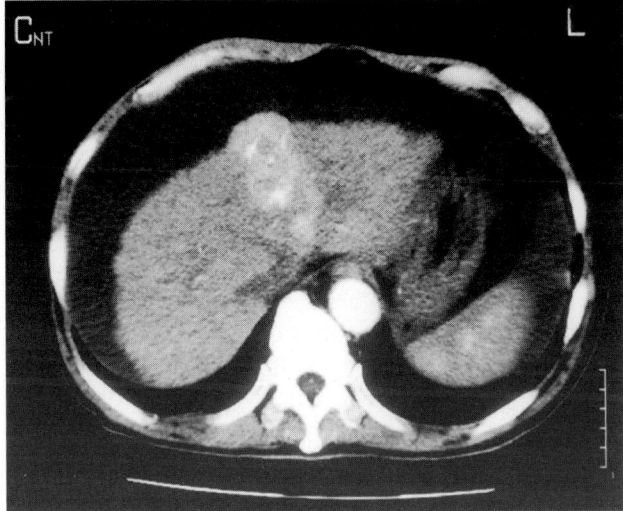

Figure 2. 58-year-old man with hepatocellular carcinoma and cirrhosis documented after liver biopsy. CT scan after injection of contrast material during arterial phase shows hyperdense mass with contour deformity of hepatic capsule.

liver. In a prospective evaluation in 50 patients undergoing liver transplantation, the detection of small HCC using lipiodol computed tomography allowed the detection of 50% of the 6 patients with cancer but only 7% of cancerous lesions [48]. In the same group of patients, the detection of small HCC by lipiodol retention on X-ray analyses of 1 cm slices of the explanted liver was fairly specific (83%) but its sensitivity (45%) was poor [49]. In another similar study performed on 72 transplanted patients, lesion by lesion analysis of the 24 HCC observed in 14 patients revealed a sensitivity of 37% with a specificity of

94% for all patients of lipiodol computed tomography [50]. Spreafico et al. [51] have shown that the sensitivity of lipiodol computed tomography for the detection of HCC depends on the size of malignancy: 90% for lesions › 2 cm and 28% for lesions ‹ 2 cm. The comparison between lipiodol computed tomography and triphasic helical CT has shown than 92% of the lesions detected by the former method were detected by the latter [52]. In this study, only patients with hypervascular HCCs were included. The other limitations of lipiodol computed tomography is the presence of false-positive diagnoses of tumor despite fair specificity, which could lead to unnecessary surgery. Dense but patchy uptake at the periphery or in the centre of the lesion may occur with haemangiomas, metastases and focal nodular hyperplasia [46, 53-55]. The tumoral necrosis induced by the injected lipiodol can also lead to false positive [56]. Finally lipiodol computed tomography appears to be an insensitive method for the detection of small HCC in livers with advanced cirrhosis.

The current task for the radiologist is to differentiate a benign regenerative nodule, a dysplastic nodule, and a dysplastic nodule containing an evolving early well-differentiated HCC. Determination between HCC and dysplastic nodules can be accomplished by the use of dual phase helical CT. Indeed, it has been demonstrated that dysplastic nodules have a predominant portal venous supply in 96% of the cases while HCC have mainly a hepatic artery supply in 94% of the cases [57]. Thus, one can hypothesise that differentiation between dysplastic nodule and an overt HCC might be made on the basis of differences in blood supply during **dual-phase** CT. However the detection of dysplastic nodule with *foci* of HCC in cirrhotic patient is a difficult issue. This small nodular lesion is characterised by i) the absence of fibrous capsule, ii) the presence of microscopic foci of HCC composed of well-differentiated tumor cells with rare architectural atypia, iii) a main portal blood supply. Therefore, its vascular pattern during dual-phase helical CT scanner, isoattenuation, is similar to the liver parenchyma which makes it impossible to be detected and differentiated. Approximately 45% of these nodules are isoattenuated or enhanced on both hepatic artery phase and portal venous phase scans. Consequently CT during early and late liver enhancement has a sensitivity of only 56% to detect dysplastic nodule with *foci* of HCC [58]. However the development of an arterial blood supply in a dysplastic nodule is a good marker of its malignant transformation. At this step of the hepatocarcinogenesis, from regenerative nodule to overt HCC, dual-phase CT has a major interest, depicting up to 95% of tumor foci [43].

Eventually, in patients being considered for major hepatic resection, it is essential to evaluate preoperatively the permeability of the portal venous system because portal vein involvement by the tumor may render the tumor unresecable or request a change in the surgical approach. The ability of contrast-enhanced CT to detect portal vein thrombus, either benign or malignant has been well-documented in the literature [59-61]. The differentiation between benign or malignant portal vein thrombus is crucial for therapeutical strategies. In a study performed on 58 cirrhotic patients, 47 with malignant and 11 with benign portal vein thrombus, identification of a main portal vein thrombus diameter greater or equal to 23 mm or neovascularity seen on CT scan was highly suggestive of malignant thrombus *(figure 3)*. The sensitivity and specificity for the CT characterisation of malignant portal vein thrombosis were 86% and 100% respectively [62]. Another study has reported that helical CT is sensitive and specific for portal venous system thrombosis [63].

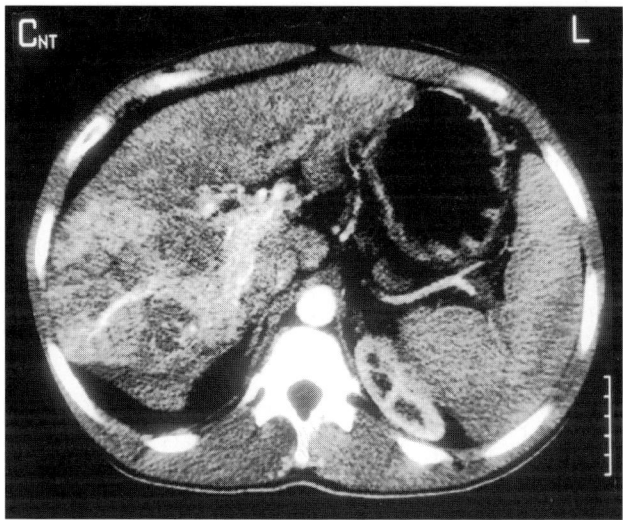

Figure 3. 35-year-old man with multifocal hepatocellular carcinoma, portal venous tumor thrombus and cirrhosis due to hepatitis B. CT scan after injection of contrast material during arterial phase shows hyperdense lesions in both right and left hepatic lobes. The portal vein is enlarged by the tumor thrombus. Linear enhancements represent tumor vessels within the thrombus. Arterioportal shunting is probably responsible for dense accumulation of contrast material in the vein (note the minimal enhancement of the spleen).

Magnetic resonance imaging

Recently, numerous technical advances have been made to improve magnetic resonance (MR) imaging of the liver. If in the past, motion artefacts have been a major source of image degradation, artefact-free MR images of the liver can now be routinely obtained in many centres. Performing the image acquisition within 15 to 30 seconds, *i.e.* within a comfortable breath-hold, can now easily control the respiratory motion artefacts. Signal intensity on T1-weighted sequences of HCC can be due to fatty change, fibrosis or haemorrhage. On T2-weighted sequences HCCs are usually hyperintense [64]. The hypervascularization of HCC is best depicted on contrast-enhanced dynamic T1-weighted sequences in the arterial phase [65]. The MR imaging protocol should also include T2-weighted sequences and dynamic contrast-enhanced MR imaging with breath-hold gradient echo sequences after gadolinium injection [66]. MR images should be acquired during the hepatic arterial phase, the portal venous phase and the equilibrium phase of liver enhancement. Global positive rates of MR imaging in patients with HCC are shown on *table II*. By comparison to biphasic helical CT, dynamic contrast-enhanced MR imaging seems to be more sensitive for the detection of small HCC foci. The detection rate of HCC smaller than 1 cm was found to be 55% for MR imaging compared to 36% for helical CT. For the detection of tumors with a diameter in the range of 1 to 2 cm, the sensitivity of dynamic MR imaging was almost identical to those of helical CT: 83% and 76% respectively [65]. Siderotic nodules, such as HCC, are characterised by their low signal in both T1- and T2-weighted spin-echo images. However, a recent study based on the comparison between thin-section MR imaging performed on fresh whole explanted livers from 30 non-Asian patients and pathological findings has challenged current concepts for the MR imaging differentiation of benign from malignant nodules in cirrhotic liver. Indeed the distinction between dysplastic nodule from HCC based on MR imaging was impossible because the signal intensity for HCC varied so much [67]. However the distinction between the two lesions may be easier if a focus of high signal intensity within a dysplastic nodule on T2-weighted images is seen. This sign is highly suspicious of early HCC, which is also termed the nodule-in nodule sign [68].

Table II. Sensitivity of magnetic resonance imaging for the detection of hepatocellular carcinoma (HCC)

References	Number of patients	Total number of HCC	Sensitivity (%)
[38]	8	32	57
[126]	15	31	63
[127]	512	43	72
[65]	49	242	62
[128]	32	37	62
[129]	23	65	53

The use of MR imaging contrast material provides additional information useful for characterisation of focal hepatic lesions, especially for the detection of liver metastases [69]. Initially most of the contrast-enhanced MR imaging examination were performed using extracellular contrast agents. Following the intravenous administration of these contrast agents, the liver undergoes four phases of enhancement as they were observed during CT: i) arterial phase which reveals lesions supplied by the hepatic arteries such as HCC, ii) portal venous phase which reveals hypovascular lesions supplied such as colorectal metastases, iii) phase of hepatic contrast enhancement (also called the equilibrium phase). During this phase, the contrast between most focal hepatic lesions and normal liver is the lowest, iv) late phase of hepatic contrast enhancement is also called the excretory phase and usually occurs 4 to 6 hours after intravenous contrast injection. Imaging at this phase is usually not routinely performed. Many new contrast agents have been developed [70]. Ferumoxide (previously known as AMI-25) is targeted to the reticuloendothelial system. It has been shown that the ability to characterise focal hepatic lesions using these agents is limited to lesions containing Kupffer cells such as focal nodular hyperplasia [71]. More recently a new class of MR imaging agent targeted to functioning hepatocytes became commercially available. Following administration of one of these new agents, such as gadolinium-BOPTA, functioning hepatocytes take up these agents and appear as regions of higher signal intensity on T1-weighted images. It has been shown that lesions containing functioning hepatocytes such as HCC and regenerating nodules take up these contrast agents and can be differentiated from non-hepatocyte-containing lesions such as liver metastases [72-76]. However the definite role of MR imaging cell-specific contrast agents for evaluation of HCC in the presence of cirrhosis is still debated. One issue raised for these cell-specific contrast agents is the reduced uptake due to the liver disease [77].

Positron emission tomography

18F-fluorodeoxyglucose (FDG) uptake allows for the estimation of glucose metabolism by cells using positron emission tomography (PET). Because there is increased glycolysis in cancer cells, whole body PET with FDG can be used to detect cancers. The difference of glucose metabolism among liver tumors and liver parenchyma results in increased accumulation of FDG in HCC [78, 79], potentially allowing differentiation between malignant and non-malignant tissue. In a study performed on 20 patients with HCC, the sensitivity of PET for the diagnosis of HCC was 55% compared to 90% for CT scanning. However PET allowed for the detection of metastases in three patients that were not seen on CT. Well-differentiated tumors and those with low tumor grades had less activity on PET and corresponding lower PET score [80]. Furthermore, PET imaging does not appear to be useful in distinguishing regenerative nodules from HCC [81]. These results must be confirmed before definitive recommendations but the usefulness of PET scan for diagnosis of HCC seems to be limited.

Screening for hepatocellular carcinoma

Screening for HCC has become, at least among hepatologists, an accepted part of the management of patients with end-stage liver disease. Patients with cirrhosis screened for HCC have an annual incidence of HCC of about 3% in Western patients and 6% in Japanese patients [82, 83]. Suggested strategies for screening have included periodic ultrasound or CT examinations or monitoring of tumor-related proteins (alpha-fetoprotein, des-gama-carboxyprothrombin) or some combination of these. Among tumors detected by surveillance, 50% to 75% were unifocal and 3 cm or less in size, and thus potentially curable. In the majority of surveillance studies, the overall surgical resection rate varied from 29% to 54% [84]. In all studies, resection was preferred to transplantation and the design did not make it possible to determine if screening influences mortality. The cost-effectiveness of screening for HCC is still debated. There are only three analyses of the cost of screening for HCC. Kang et al. [85], in a study of HBV carriers, concluded that using AFP and ultrasound screening yearly would detect 90% of early tumors at a cost of US $11800 each. In a large mass screening study of 8,090 Japanese patients at risk for HCC, 91 tumors were detected (1.1%) at a cost of US $25000 per tumor [86]. In neither of these cost-benefit analyses were postscreening diagnostic costs included, nor was the cost per year of life gained reported. The third study was based on theoretical model, *i.e.* decision analysis model representing the natural history of cirrhosis and the continuing risk of developing cancer [87]. For most patients seen in the daily practice, screening based on ultrasound and AFP performed every 6 months provide negligible benefits in life expectancy (< 3 months). The cost-effectiveness ratio of systematic surveillance ranges between US $48000 and US $284000 for each additional life-year gained, more than other common medical practices. For well-targeted patients with the longest reported-related survival rate, the cost-effectiveness ratio ranges between US $26000 and US $55000 for each additional life-year gained. However, the authors did not consider orthotopic liver transplantation as a therapeutic option in their model. Therefore, before recommending such expensive surveillance programmes, it is mandatory to develop reliable therapeutic options with a clear-cut benefit in terms of survival.

Imaging and staging of liver metastases

Metastases represent the most common hepatic malignancies. Virtually every primary tumor may disseminate to the liver but the most common primaries are colon and rectum, stomach, pancreas, breast and lung. In many patients suffering from neoplastic disease, liver involvement is a major determinant of survival and its discovery may lead to significant changes in the management of the disease. Although clinical examination and disturbances of liver function tests may be indicative of advanced liver tumors, the diagnosis of liver metastases at an earlier stage is almost entirely dependent on imaging. In this context, the success of imaging depends not only on its ability to resolve small liver lesions, but also on its ability to characterise these lesions and to distinguish between metastases and non-malignant lesions such as cysts, haemangiomas, biliary hamartomas, focal fatty changes... Once the diagnosis of liver metastases has been established, the possibility of hepatic resection should always be considered in the particular setting of colorectal primaries. A careful selection of patients amenable to surgery is crucial to avoid unnecessary operations. Again, this selection relies on imaging and requires accurate determination of the extent and location of metastastic lesions, as well as of the relationship of lesions to major venous structures. Imaging has also a major role in the evaluation of treatment efficacy in patients with unresectable colorectal liver metastases or metastases from other primaries, treated with chemotherapy. Ultrasonography (US), computed tomography (CT) and magnetic resonance imaging (MRI) are the three main techniques available to the clinician today. However, technological advances together with the development of contrast agent material has allowed for a refinement and a continuing improvement on imaging protocols. Because of a concomitant increase of medical expenditure, analysis of the imaging modalities has become necessary to address the issue of the most cost-effective strategies in these three circumstances.

Screening for liver metastases

Percutaneous ultrasonography offers a rapid, non-invasive, and relatively inexpensive method for screening patients for liver metastases. It is widely used as the first-line investigation in this situation and is recommended by some authors in the regular follow-up of patients after curative resection of colorectal cancer. Its sensitivity is frequently overestimated and quoted as 80% to 85%. In fact, the sensitivity of US in the detection of individual lesions, as assessed in studies with surgical or pathological correlation, is much lower and highly dependent on the size of the lesions [88]. Difficulties with US include the fact that lesions may be missed for operator-dependent or perceptual reasons and that the differences in echogenicity between metastases and the surrounding liver may be low (so-called isoechoic lesions). Several techniques have been developed or are under investigation in an attempt to improve the sensitivity of US for the detection of liver metastases, especially of centimeter or subcentimeter lesions. Conventional spectral or color Doppler sonography, performed during the same exploration, may provide additional information in depicting tumor's vascularity [32, 89]. Power Doppler sonography, which is based on the total integrated Doppler power spectrum, would be even more accurate, because of its superiority over color Doppler to detect slow blood flow [90]. Signal enhancing contrast material are microbubble agents that interact in various complex ways with the ultrasound beam after intravenous administration during US [91]. This interaction results in a Doppler enhancement and allows for a better detection of smaller lesions. Stimulated acoustic emission and pulse-inversion imaging modes after administration of microbubble agents produce a dramatic increase in the conspicuity of liver metastases and offers new promising potentialities [92, 93]. The analysis of US images obtained at two centre frequencies is another promising technique that may improve both lesion detectability and characterisation [94].

Because of its cost, the radiation induced and the need of intravenous administration of contrast material, computed tomography (CT) is usually considered inappropriate for screening purposes and performed only in patients with non informative or doubtful US exploration. Since conventional CT consists in obtaining consecutive scans during separate periods of respiratory failure, unequal breath holding may lead to data gasps between successive sections and eventually hamper depiction of focal hepatic lesions. The detection rate of liver metastases may be improved by the combination of conventional unenhanced CT with incremental bolus dynamic CT and scan during the time of peak hepatic parenchymal enhancement, which occurs during the portal venous-dominant phase (PVP) of the contrast enhancement curve [95]. Helical CT provides many theoretical advantages over incremental CT for detecting malignant hepatic tumors, including reduced or eliminated respiratory misregistration, imaging during the optimal window of contrast enhancement for maximal lesion conspicuity, and the ability to reconstruct axial images at arbitrary intervals to better centre the sections over focal lesions [96]. Moreover, the introduction of helical technology has allowed for a dramatic reduction in the time required to scan the liver to the point that the entire liver can be imaged two times after intravenous administration of a single bolus of contrast material, once during the early hepatic arterial-dominant phase (HAP) and again during the portal venous-dominant phase of contrast enhancement. This has led to the popularisation of dual-or triple phase imaging of the liver that exploits the dual blood supply to liver parenchyma and the inherent differences in blood supply to liver tumor and liver parenchyma. However, the optimal CT technique for the evaluation of liver metastases has been the subject of considerable investigations and controversies. Because imaging during PVP reveals the greatest tumors in patients with hypovascular liver neoplasms which enhance only minimally, and because most metastatic neoplasms of the liver are hypovascular, the PVP acquisition became the universally accepted routine procedure *(figure 4)* [97]. Although the addition of HAP and noncontrast-phase (NCP) imaging to PVP acquisition has been demonstrated to be beneficial for the detection of hepatocarcinoma, their relative benefit is less convincing in patients with hypervascular liver metastases (such as metastases from neuroendocrine and carcinoid tumors, pheochromocytoma, melanoma, renal cell carcinoma...) [98-100], and even more questionable in patients with hypovascular metastases and notably colorectal primaries. The issue of the contribution afforded by HAP and NCP images is important to address because multi-phase imaging has economic implications, including higher doses or rates (or both) of contrast material administration, increased film costs, additional scanner and technologist time, and increased burden on the X-ray tube. An additional factor is the overall increase in patient radiation exposure.

Preoperative assessment of patients considered for hepatic surgery

Complete surgical resection of hepatic colorectal metastases has been demonstrated to result in long-term survival in more than one third of patients [101]. In spite of significant advances in systemic chemotherapy, surgery remains the sole potentially curative treatment

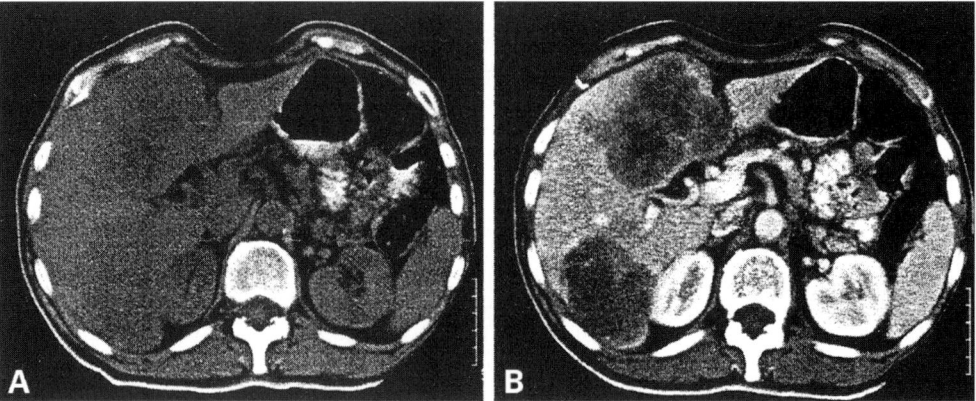

Figure 4. 48-year-old women with colon cancer liver metastases. (A) Unenhanced helical CT scan shows two liver tumors located in segments IV and VI, whose density is only slightly different from that of surrounding parenchyma. (B) Helical CT scan obtained during the portal venous-dominant phase of contrast enhancement shows the two metastases which enhance only minimally compared with normal surrounding parenchyma. The significant improvement of lesion-to-liver contrast allows for a markedly better visualisation and demarcation of these lesions.

in the context of metastatic disease and should always be considered in this situation. Unfortunately, up to now, surgical treatment could only be offered to approximately 10% of the patients who present with metastases from colorectal cancer. More recently, favourable results have also been reported with surgery following downstaging of initially nonresectable liver metastases with effective chemotherapy regimen [102]. These data, together with improvements in hepatic oncologic surgery and possible association with cryotherapy or radiofrequency ablation, have resulted in both an increase in the number of candidates for potential hepatic resection and a decrease in operative mortality and morbidity. In any case, careful preoperative selection of patients through the use of appropriate imaging studies is crucial to avoid unnecessary surgical explorations that may have detrimental effect on quality of life and to plan the type of surgical resection necessary in resectable patients.

- **Computed tomography during arterial portography (CTAP)**, whose sensitivity for the detection of focal hepatic lesions ranges from 81% to 94%, was widely accepted as the most accurate technique for preoperative assessment of patients being considered for hepatic resection. This method is based on the selective delivery of contrast medium to the portal venous system through an angiographic catheter placed into the superior mesenteric artery by means of trans-femoral approach, without distribution or dilution with the central blood volume. Hepatic neoplasms, whose blood supply derives mainly from hepatic artery, remain unenhanced during the portal and parenchymal phases of contrast material distribution and are therefore detected as hypoattenuating areas. Rapid acquisition after injection is mandatory, because recirculation of contrast medium to the systemic circulation will result in diminished contrast differences between neoplasm and normal parenchyma. Recent introduction of helical CT, which allows for scanning the entire liver within a narrow time window during a single breath-hold sequence, has resulted in an improvement in sensitivity, due to high vascular and parenchyma enhancement and lack of respiratory motion [103-106]. However, in spite of this progress, the accuracy of the technique for the depiction of metastases smaller than 1 cm remains poor, with a sensitivity of 52% in a recent published multiobserver study [106]. The need for vascular catheterization makes CTAP an invasive procedure and may explain some technical failures and complications. A relatively high false-positive rate, mainly related to perfusion abnormalities and perfusion defects, is another disadvantage of CTAP, that should lead to interpret findings of this investigation alone with some caution [107]. The frequency of these perfusion abnormalities is depending on imaging technique, especially on the volume and the injection rate of contrast material and on the scanning delay after administration [108]. Dual-phase protocol may also limit perfusion artefacts [105], and prior intra-arterial injection of vasodilator may be beneficial in increasing portal blood flow and hence in improving homogeneity of hepatic enhancement. It is therefore critical to respect an optimised and standardised protocol in order to achieve the best accuracy. Some of note, studies suggest that optimised PVP intravenous contrast-enhanced helical CT may be as accurate as CTAP for the diagnosis of liver metastases and may represent a valuable alternative in the context of preoperative work-up, but this deserves further comparative evaluation [97].

- Although conventional nonenhanced MRI imaging is not suitable for the preoperative assessment of patients with potentially resectable colorectal liver metastases [38], recent advances in the field of MRI have lead to revisit its role in this situation. In fact, the development of newer sequence designs and the use of several contrast agents have yielded promising results for the detection and the characterisation of focal liver lesions. Improvements in gradient technology have allowed for the development of rapid pulse sequences. These different techniques dramatically reduce image acquisition time compared with conventional T1- and T2-weighted spin-echo acquisitions and are highly suitable for breath-hold imaging, which considerably lessens artefacts secondary to gross physiologic motion (respiration, bowel peristalsis, cardiac pulsation). Breath-hold gradient-echo sequences for T1-weighted acquisitions was first described [109] and the capabilities for breath-hold T2-weighted acquisitions have more recently emerged (multishot fast imaging techniques such as fast spin-echo - FSE -, inversion-recovery fast SE - IR FSE -and fast gradient SE imaging and single shot techniques such as half-Fourier-single-shot-fast-SE and echo-planar - EP - imaging) [110]. Ultra-fast single shot sequences may be particularly useful in patients who are unable to achieve sufficient breath hold. These sequences may be associated with fat-saturation technique and contrast enhancement. Several studies have confirmed that detection, localisation and characterisation of liver lesions were significantly better and more confidently performed with breath-hold MR imaging. Moreover, images are generally obtained with high tissue contrast, providing an excellent lesion conspicuousness. Simultaneously, several contrast agents have been developed in an attempt to enhance the contrast between hepatic focal lesions and surrounding parenchyma and eventually to improve the diagnostic potential of MRI. Intravenous administration of gadolinium-based contrast material has been first investigated and breath-hold T1-weighted gradient-echo (GRE) sequence acquired during the hepatic arterial dominant phase of gadolinium enhancement has been recently demonstrated to have a high diagnostic accuracy with a sensitivity similar to that of spiral CTAP for lesion detection and a greater specificity [111, 112]. Tissue-specific agents, including superparamagnetic iron oxide (SPIO) particles and hepatobiliary agents such as gadolinium benzyloxypropionictetraacetate (BOPTA) and manganese DPDP, also achieved promising results [69, 72, 74, 106, 113, 114]. The former are taken up by the reticuloendothelial system and induce a selective signal loss of healthy liver, whereas the latter are primarily taken up by hepatocytes with subsequent prolonged enhancement of liver parenchyma. As a whole, the major strength of MRI over CTAP is a higher specificity due to a better recognition of perfusion defects together with a better characterisation of lesions approximately 1 cm in diameter. The conjunction of the high diagnostic performance of optimised MRI with its non invasive nature and substantially lesser radiation exposure and charges than CTAP [111] are compelling reasons to adopt this imaging modality over CTAP in the preoperative work-up of patients with potentially resectable colorectal liver metastases. In a prospective study using intraoperative ultrasonography as the standard of reference for pathological proof in 17 patients, the accuracy of CTAP, unenhanced MRI and ferumoxides-enhanced MR imaging for the detection of hepatic metastases was 0.925, 0.908 and 0.951 respectively [69]. However, it is noteworthy that the accuracy of MRI is highly dependent upon imaging parameters and protocols used and that its sensitivity for the detection of subcentimeter lesions is still disappointing, in the region of 50%, even with optimised procedure [106]. The different techniques available today should be compared with each other in order to define the best cost-effective method that should be routinely used in a reproducible fashion and recommended in this situation and to answer several questions: which sequence and imaging parameters should be used: should several sequences be combined? In which planes should image acquisition be performed (transverse, coronal)? What is the optimised timing for contrast medium administration?

- **Intraoperative ultrasonography (IOUS)** has been advocated as an important aid in the decision-making process because it can depict small metastatic nodules that cannot be detected with conventional imaging modalities. In fact, in spite of its high sensitivity and specificity for the diagnosis of liver metastases, its impact on treatment strategy and surgical management is probably marginal, especially in patients having being submitted to a careful preoperative evaluation by means of a highly sensitive technique such as helical CTAP or optimised MRI [115, 116]. Moreover, IOUS, which requires a wide hepatic exposure, cannot prevent the careful preoperative evaluation to assess the feasibility of hepatic resection and to avoid unnecessary surgical explorations. On the other hand, IOUS is widely accepted as an important peroperative aid to perform safe hepatic resection because anatomic vascular structures (hepatic veins and portal branches) are very well outlined and the extent of the disease is well delineated. IOUS and CTAP or MRI should therefore be considered as non-competitors but complementary techniques. IOUS is also crucial during cryotherapy and radiofrequency ablation to ensure a proper position of the probes into the centre of the lesions and to monitor tumor ablation [117]. Recently, laparoscopic ultrasound probes have been developed and laparoscopic liver examination with ultrasonography during staging laparoscopy have been proposed but this remains investigational [118, 119].

A special mention should be done about imaging of the liver metastases of carcinoid and neuroendocrine tumors. US, CT and MRI remain the cornerstones for the investigation of these liver metastases and both HAP and NCP images have been demonstrated to provide added value compared with PVP images during helical CT examination [100]. Moreover, because a vast majority of these tumors display a high density of somatostatin receptors, somatostatin receptor scintigraphy using 111In-DTPA-D-Phe1 octreotide (Octreoscan) has been proposed to assess tumor spread. It appeared to have a high sensitivity and specificity for tumor localisation and provides additional information about the somatostatin receptor status. The limited spatial resolution of somatostatin receptor scintigraphy means that it rarely shows liver lesions undetectable on CT or MRI although extrahepatic disease is often demonstrated more effectively by somatostatin receptor scintigraphy than by anatomical techniques. Somatostatin receptor scintigraphy plays therefore a key role in the staging and therapeutic decision making processes and should always be performed in patients with liver metastases before hepatectomy is considered in order to identify candidates suitable for resection [120-122].

Follow-up of patients while on chemotherapy

Besides detection of liver metastases, periodic evaluation of the size of the lesions in patients treated with chemotherapy is another important issue. In fact, some of the largests and most well-circumscribed lesions present in a given patient (further referred to as "target lesions" or "indicator lesions") should be selected on pre-treatment imaging and further measured at intervals of 4 to 8 weeks while on treatment. Measurement of all target lesions in two perpendicular axes, whose product is proportional to lesions areas, is usually retained although some authors have advocated using uni- or three-dimensional methods. In any case, these measurements are important since decisions on whether to continue, suspend or alter chemotherapy are based on interval changes in size of target lesions as evaluated on serial imaging examinations. It is therefore crucial to use the imaging technique providing the more reproducible measurements from examination to examination. US is usually considered not suitable for reliable detection of changes over time and would not allow anyway for retrospective reviews. Although there has been relatively little attention given to the optimal method of measuring individual colorectal or other type of hypovascular liver metastases, the current radiological practice is to compare serial postcontrast CT-scans with each other. Because the size of liver lesions are so dependent on scanning timing, it is important to perform CT-scanning during the same phase of contrast material enhancement. Otherwise an artefactual decrease or increase in lesion size can occur, which gives a false impression of lesion regression or progression. Moreover, serial follow-up of hepatic hypovascular metastases with CT scans obtained after the administration of contrast material may not be the optimal approach. In fact, diffusion of contrast material into the extravascular space of the tumor may decrease liver-to-lesion contrast and may eventually lead to partial or complete disappearance of the tumor [123]. Several authors have suggested that non-enhanced images provide tumor measurement more accurate and more consistent from study to study and that precontrast imaging is a better way to follow the size of liver metastases but this remains to be demonstrated. Ideally, post-contrast scanning should still be performed in addition to pre-contrast imaging to optimise the detection of new lesions.

Conclusions and perspectives

The comparison of the performance of different imaging strategies for the diagnosis and the assessment of liver metastatic disease is made difficult by the huge variety of imaging procedures depending upon the hardware and the imaging protocols used. Furthermore, continuing advances in contrast agents and imaging technology gives the possibility of developing new procedures, and further improvements are anticipated in the near future that could modify the current radiological practice *(figure 5)*. This multiplicity of imaging procedures results in a large variation in the cost of imaging strategies. However, only very few data on cost-efficacy are available in the radiological literature and studies are warranted to identify the strategy achieving the most favorable cost effective relation. Moreover, although current imaging is very successful when considering liver metastases larger than 1 cm, it is relatively poor for smaller lesions. In fact, the sensitivity of optimised imaging methods for the depiction of subcentimeters lesions remains in the range of 50% when surgery with palpation and intraoperative ultrasound is used as the gold standard. Improvements in the earlier detection of metastases will probably require a fundamentally different approach than that of conventional anatomical methods. It was recently suggested that positron emission tomography using FDG-PET has a high accuracy to diagnose liver metastatic involvement in various neoplastic conditions. In combination with CT scan, it may provide additional diagnostic information by assessing the metabolic status and benign or malignant characteristic of undetermined lesions, but prospective studies are mandatory to determine the optimum role of PET in the management of patients with liver metastases [124]. At the present time, new radionuclide or Doppler perfusion methods are available to detect the modification of the ratio of arterial to portal inflow (hepatic perfusion index) that develop shortly after metastastic seeding in the liver. The identification of this abnormal liver perfusion was found to be more sensitive than conventional imaging techniques in detecting metastatic disease confirmed at surgery and also in identifying those patients most likely to develop metastases subsequently [125]. It represent a new promising approach to detect early occult hepatic micrometastases.

✔ Percutaneous ultrasonography (US) remains the imaging choice procedure for screening patients for liver metastases.

✔ The initial evaluation of hypovascular liver metastases is based on helical computed tomography during the portal venous-dominant phase of contrast enhancement.

✔ Magnetic resonance (MR) imaging using newer sequence designs and contrast enhancement tends to challenge computed tomography during arterial portography (CTAP) for the preoperative assessment of patients with potentially resectable colorectal liver metastases.

✔ Intraoperative ultrasonography (IOUS) is complementary to preoperative imaging work-up in patients considered for surgical resection of hepatic metastases.

✔ Follow-up of patients treated with chemotherapy is based on serial helical computed tomography (CT) examinations.

✔ Careful attention should be given to continuing advances in imaging technology, as they could lead to modifications in the current radiological practice in a near future.

Figure 5. Current imaging strategy for liver metastases.

*References

1. Weinstein MC, Stason WB. Foundations of cost-effectiveness analysis for health and medical practices. *N Engl J Med* 1977; 296: 716-21.
2. Neumann PJ, Stone PW, Chapman RH, Sandberg EA, Bell CM. The quality of reporting in published cost-utility analyses, 1976-1997. *Ann Intern Med* 2000; 132: 964-72.
3. Bosch FX, Ribes J, Borras J. Epidemiology of primary liver cancer. *Semin Liver Dis* 1999; 19: 271-85.
4. El-Serag HB, Mason AC. Rising incidence of hepatocellular carcinoma in the United States. *N Engl J Med* 1999; 340: 745-50.
5. Deuffic S, Poynard T, Buffat L, Valleron AJ. Trends in primary liver cancer [letter]. *Lancet* 1998; 351: 5.
6. McPeake JR, O'Grady JG, Zaman S, Portmann B, Wight DG, Tan KC, Calne RY, et al. Liver transplantation for primary hepatocellular carcinoma: tumor size and number determine outcome. *J Hepatol* 1993; 18: 226-34.
7. Penn I. Hepatic transplantation for primary and metastatic cancers of the liver. *Surgery* 1991; 110: 726-34.
8. Bismuth H, Chiche L, Adam R, Castaing D, Diamond T, Dennison A. Liver resection versus transplantation for hepatocellular carcinoma in cirrhotic patients. *Ann Surg* 1993; 218: 145-51.
9. Belghiti J. Resection of hepatocellular carcinoma complicating cirrhosis. *Br J Surg* 1991; 78: 257-8.
10. Kanematsu T, Matsumata T, Takenaka K, Yoshida Y, Higashi H, Sugimachi K. Clinical management of recurrent hepatocellular carcinoma after primary resection. *Br J Surg* 1988; 75: 203-6.
11. Theise ND. Macroregenerative (dysplastic) nodules and hepatocarcinogenesis: theoretical and clinical considerations. *Semin Liver Dis* 1995; 15: 360-71.
12. Mazzaferro V, Regalia E, Doci R, Andreola S, Pulvirenti A, Bozzetti F, Montalto F, et al. Liver transplantation for the treatment of small hepatocellular carcinomas in patients with cirrhosis. *N Engl J Med* 1996; 334: 693-9.
13. Party IW. Terminology of nodular hepatocellular lesions. *Hepatology* 1995; 22: 983-93.
14. Hytiroglou P, Theise ND, Schwartz M, Mor E, Miller C, Thung SN. Macroregenerative nodules in a series of adult cirrhotic liver explants: issues of classification and nomenclature. *Hepatology* 1995; 21: 703-8.
15. Choi BI, Takayasu K, Han MC. Small hepatocellular carcinomas and associated nodular lesions of the liver: pathology, pathogenesis, and imaging findings. *AJR Am J Roentgenol* 1993; 160: 1177-87.
16. Winter TCr, Takayasu K, Muramatsu Y, Furukawa H, Wakao F, Koga H, Sakamoto M, et al. Early advanced hepatocellular carcinoma: evaluation of CT and MR appearance with pathologic correlation. *Radiology* 1994; 192: 379-87.
17. Colombo M. Hepatocellular carcinoma in cirrhotics. *Semin Liver Dis* 1993; 13: 374-83.
18. Okuda K, Ohtsuki T, Obata H, Tomimatsu M, Okazaki N, Hasegawa H, Nakajima Y, et al. Natural history of hepatocellular carcinoma and prognosis in relation to treatment. Study of 850 patients. *Cancer* 1985; 56: 918-28.
19. Kubota K, Makuuchi M, Kusaka K, Kobayashi T, Miki K, Hasegawa K, Harihara Y, et al. Measurement of liver volume and hepatic functional reserve as a guide to decision-making in resectional surgery for hepatic tumors. *Hepatology* 1997; 26: 1176-81.
20. Lo CM, Lai EC, Liu CL, Fan ST, Wong J. Laparoscopy and laparoscopic ultrasonography avoid exploratory laparotomy in patients with hepatocellular carcinoma. *Ann Surg* 1998; 227: 527-32.
21. Choi BI, Park JH, Kim BH, Kim SH, Han MC, Kim CW. Small hepatocellular carcinoma: detection with sonography, computed tomography (CT), angiography and Lipiodol-CT. *Br J Radiol* 1989; 62: 897-903.
22. Sheu JC, Sung JL, Chen DS, Yu JY, Wang TH, Su CT, Tsang YM. Ultrasonography of small hepatic tumors using high-resolution linear-array real-time instruments. *Radiology* 1984; 150: 797-802.

23. Clarke MP, Kane RA, Steele G, Jr., Hamilton ES, Ravikumar TS, Onik G, Clouse ME. Prospective comparison of preoperative imaging and intraoperative ultrasonography in the detection of liver tumors. *Surgery* 1989; 106: 849-55.
24. Gazelle GS, Haaga JR. Hepatic neoplasms: surgically relevant segmental anatomy and imaging techniques. *AJR Am J Roentgenol* 1992; 158: 1015-8.
25. Kudo M, Hirasa M, Takakuwa H, Ibuki Y, Fujimi K, Miyamura M, Tomita S, *et al*. Small hepatocellular carcinomas in chronic liver disease: detection with SPECT. *Radiology* 1986; 159: 697-703.
26. Ros PR, Murphy BJ, Buck JL, Olmedilla G, Goodman Z. Encapsulated hepatocellular carcinoma: radiologic findings and pathologic correlation. *Gastrointest Radiol* 1990; 15: 233-7.
27. Tanaka S, Kitamura T, Ohshima A, Umeda K, Okuda S, Ohtani T, Tatsuta M, *et al*. Diagnostic accuracy of ultrasonography for hepatocellular carcinoma. *Cancer* 1986; 58: 344-7.
28. Tanaka S, Kitamura T, Nakanishi K, Okuda S, Kojima J, Fujimoto I. Recent advances in ultrasonographic diagnosis of hepatocellular carcinoma. *Cancer* 1989; 63: 1313-7.
29. Japan LCSGo. Primary liver cancer in Japan. Clinicopathologic features and results of surgical treatment. *Ann Surg* 1990; 211: 277-87.
30. Mathieu D, Guinet C, Bouklia-Hassane A, Vasile N. Hepatic vein involvement in hepatocellular carcinoma. *Gastrointest Radiol* 1988; 13: 55-60.
31. Dodd GDr, Memel DS, Baron RL, Eichner L, Santiguida LA. Portal vein thrombosis in patients with cirrhosis: does sonographic detection of intrathrombus flow allow differentiation of benign and malignant thrombus? *AJR Am J Roentgenol* 1995; 165: 573-7.
32. Nino-Murcia M, Ralls PW, Jeffrey RB, Jr., Johnson M. Color flow Doppler characterization of focal hepatic lesions. *AJR Am J Roentgenol* 1992; 159: 1195-7.
33. Reinhold C, Hammers L, Taylor CR, Quedens-Case CL, Holland CK, Taylor KJ. Characterization of focal hepatic lesions with duplex sonography: findings in 198 patients. AJR *Am J Roentgenol* 1995; 164: 1131-5.
34. Tanaka S, Kitamra T, Fujita M, Kasugai H, Inoue A, Ishiguro S. Small hepatocellular carcinoma: differentiation from adenomatous hyperplastic nodule with color Doppler flow imaging. *Radiology* 1992; 182: 161-5.
35. Nagasue N, Yukaya H, Ogawa Y, Sasaki Y, Chang YC, Niimi K. Clinical experience with 118 hepatic resections for hepatocellular carcinoma. *Surgery* 1986; 99: 694-701.
36. Miller WJ, Federle MP, Campbell WL. Diagnosis and staging of hepatocellular carcinoma: comparison of CT and sonography in 36 liver transplantation patients. *AJR Am J Roentgenol* 1991; 157: 303-6.
37. Dodd GDd, Miller WJ, Baron RL, Skolnick ML, Campbell WL. Detection of malignant tumors in end-stage cirrhotic livers: efficacy of sonography as a screening technique. *AJR Am J Roentgenol* 1992; 159: 727-33.
38. Heiken JP, Weyman PJ, Lee JK, Balfe DM, Picus D, Brunt EM, Flye MW. Detection of focal hepatic masses: prospective evaluation with CT, delayed CT, CT during arterial portography, and MR imaging. *Radiology* 1989; 171: 47-51.
39. Vassiliades VG, Foley WD, Alarcon J, Lawson T, Erickson S, Kneeland JB, Steinberg HV, *et al*. Hepatic metastases: CT versus MR imaging at 1.5T. *Gastrointest Radiol* 1991; 16: 159-63.
40. Miller WJ, Baron RL, Dodd GDr, Federle MP. Malignancies in patients with cirrhosis: CT sensitivity and specificity in 200 consecutive transplant patients. *Radiology* 1994; 193: 645-50.
41. Baron RL. Understanding and optimizing use of contrast material for CT of the liver. *AJR Am J Roentgenol* 1994; 163: 323-31.
42. Baron RL, Oliver JHr, Dodd GDr, Nalesnik M, Holbert BL, Carr B. Hepatocellular carcinoma: evaluation with biphasic, contrast-enhanced, helical CT. *Radiology* 1996; 199: 505-11.
43. Hollett MD, Jeffrey RB, Jr., Nino-Murcia M, Jorgensen MJ, Harris DP. Dual-phase helical CT of the liver: value of arterial phase scans in the detection of small (< or = 1.5 cm) malignant hepatic neoplasms. *AJR Am J Roentgenol* 1995; 164: 879-84.

44. van Leeuwen MS, Noordzij J, Feldberg MA, Hennipman AH, Doornewaard H. Focal liver lesions: characterization with triphasic spiral CT. *Radiology* 1996; 201: 327-36.
45. Ueda K, Matsui O, Kawamori Y, Nakanuma Y, Kadoya M, Yoshikawa J, Gabata T, *et al*. Hypervascular hepatocellular carcinoma: evaluation of hemodynamics with dynamic CT during hepatic arteriography. *Radiology* 1998; 206: 161-6.
46. Ngan H. Lipiodol computerized tomography: how sensitive and specific is the technique in the diagnosis of hepatocellular carcinoma? *Br J Radiol* 1990; 63: 771-5.
47. Takayasu K, Moriyama N, Muramatsu Y, Makuuchi M, Hasegawa H, Okazaki N, Hirohashi S. The diagnosis of small hepatocellular carcinomas: efficacy of various imaging procedures in 100 patients. *AJR Am J Roentgenol* 1990; 155: 49-54.
48. Saada J, Bhattacharya S, Dhillon AP, Dick R, Burroughs AK, Rolles K, Davidson BR. Detection of small hepatocellular carcinomas in cirrhotic livers using iodised oil computed tomography. *Gut* 1997; 41: 404-7.
49. Bhattacharya S, Dhillon AP, Rees J, Savage K, Saada J, Burroughs A, Rolles K, *et al*. Small hepatocellular carcinomas in cirrhotic explant livers: identification by macroscopic examination and lipiodol localization. *Hepatology* 1997; 25: 613-8.
50. Bizollon T, Rode A, Bancel B, Gueripel V, Ducerf C, Baulieux J, Trepo C. Diagnostic value and tolerance of Lipiodol-computed tomography for the detection of small hepatocellular carcinoma: correlation with pathologic examination of explanted livers. *J Hepatol* 1998; 28: 491-6.
51. Spreafico C, Marchiano A, Mazzaferro V, Frigerio LF, Regalia E, Lanocita R, Patelli G, *et al*. Hepatocellular carcinoma in patients who undergo liver transplantation: sensitivity of CT with iodized oil. *Radiology* 1997; 203: 457-60.
52. Choi BI, Lee HJ, Han JK, Choi DS, Seo JB, Han MC. Detection of hypervascular nodular hepatocellular carcinomas: value of triphasic helical CT compared with iodized-oil CT. *AJR Am J Roentgenol* 1997; 168: 219-24.
53. Yumoto Y, Jinno K, Tokuyama K, Araki Y, Ishimitsu T, Maeda H, Konno T, *et al*. Hepatocellular carcinoma detected by iodized oil. *Radiology* 1985; 154: 19-24.
54. Maki S, Konno T, Maeda H. Image enhancement in computerized tomography for sensitive diagnosis of liver cancer and semiquantitation of tumor selective drug targeting with oily contrast medium. *Cancer* 1985; 56: 751-7.
55. Bruneton JN, Kerboul P, Grimaldi C, Normand F, Balu-Maestro C, Rampal P, Delmont J. Hepatic intraarterial lipiodol: technique, semiologic patterns, and value for hepatic tumors. *Gastrointest Radiol* 1988; 13: 45-51.
56. Arnold MM, Kreel L, Wallace AC, Li AK. Distribution of Lipiodol and evidence for tumor necrosis in hepatocellular carcinoma. *Am J Clin Pathol* 1992; 97: 405-10.
57. Matsui O, Kadoya M, Kameyama T, Yoshikawa J, Takashima T, Nakanuma Y, Unoura M, *et al*. Benign and malignant nodules in cirrhotic livers: distinction based on blood supply. *Radiology* 1991; 178: 493-7.
58. Takayasu K, Furukawa H, Wakao F, Muramatsu Y, Abe H, Terauchi T, Winter TCr, *et al*. CT diagnosis of early hepatocellular carcinoma: sensitivity, findings, and CT-pathologic correlation. *AJR Am J Roentgenol* 1995; 164: 885-90.
59. Martin K, Balfe DM, Lee JK. Computed tomography of portal vein thrombosis: unusual appearances and pitfalls in diagnosis. *J Comput Assist Tomogr* 1989; 13: 811-6.
60. Marn CS, Francis IR. CT of portal venous occlusion. *AJR Am J Roentgenol* 1992; 159: 717-26.
61. Parvey HR, Raval B, Sandler CM. Portal vein thrombosis: imaging findings. *AJR Am J Roentgenol* 1994; 162: 77-81.
62. Tublin ME, Dodd GDr, Baron RL. Benign and malignant portal vein thrombosis: differentiation by CT characteristics. *AJR Am J Roentgenol* 1997; 168: 719-23.

63. Kuszyk BS, Osterman FA, Jr., Venbrux AC, Heath DG, Urban BA, Smith PA, Fishman EK. Portal venous system thrombosis: helical CT angiography before transjugular intrahepatic portosystemic shunt creation. *Radiology* 1998; 206: 179-86.
64. Rummeny E, Weissleder R, Stark DD, Saini S, Compton CC, Bennett W, Hahn PF, *et al*. Primary liver tumors: diagnosis by MR imaging. *AJR Am J Roentgenol* 1989; 152: 63-72.
65. Oi H, Murakami T, Kim T, Matsushita M, Kishimoto H, Nakamura H. Dynamic MR imaging and early-phase helical CT for detecting small intrahepatic metastases of hepatocellular carcinoma. *AJR Am J Roentgenol* 1996; 166: 369-74.
66. Semelka RC, Willms AB, Brown MA, Brown ED, Finn JP. Comparison of breath-hold T1-weighted MR sequences for imaging of the liver. *J Magn Reson Imaging* 1994; 4: 759-65.
67. Earls JP, Theise ND, Weinreb JC, DeCorato DR, Krinsky GA, Rofsky NM, Mizrachi H, *et al*. Dysplastic nodules and hepatocellular carcinoma: thin-section MR imaging of explanted cirrhotic livers with pathologic correlation. *Radiology* 1996; 201: 207-14.
68. Mitchell DG, Rubin R, Siegelman ES, Burk DL, Jr., Rifkin MD. Hepatocellular carcinoma within siderotic regenerative nodules: appearance as a nodule within a nodule on MR images. *Radiology* 1991; 178: 101-3.
69. Seneterre E, Taourel P, Bouvier Y, Pradel J, Van Beers B, Daures JP, Pringot J, *et al*. Detection of hepatic metastases: ferumoxides-enhanced MR imaging versus unenhanced MR imaging and CT during arterial portography. *Radiology* 1996; 200: 785-92.
70. Mahfouz AE, Hamm B, Taupitz M. Contrast agents for MR imaging of the liver: a clinical overview. *Eur Radiol* 1997; 7: 507-13.
71. Denys A, Arrive L, Servois V, Dubray B, Najmark D, Sibert A, Menu Y. Hepatic tumors: detection and characterization at 1-T MR imaging enhanced with AMI-25. *Radiology* 1994; 193: 665-9.
72. Hamm B, Vogl TJ, Branding G, Schnell B, Taupitz M, Wolf KJ, Lissner J. Focal liver lesions: MR imaging with MnDPDP-initial clinical results in 40 patients. *Radiology* 1992; 182: 167-74.
73. Liou J, Lee JK, Borrello JA, Brown JJ. Differentiation of hepatomas from nonhepatomatous masses: use of MnDPDP-enhanced MR images. *Magn Reson Imaging* 1994; 12: 71-9.
74. Vogl TJ, Kummel S, Hammerstingl R, Schellenbeck M, Schumacher G, Balzer T, Schwarz W, *et al*. Liver tumors: comparison of MR imaging with Gd-EOB-DTPA and Gd-DTPA. *Radiology* 1996; 200: 59-67.
75. Reimer P, Rummeny EJ, Daldrup HE, Hesse T, Balzer T, Tombach B, Peters PE. Enhancement characteristics of liver metastases, hepatocellular carcinomas, and hemangiomas with Gd-EOB-DTPA: preliminary results with dynamic MR imaging. *Eur Radiol* 1997; 7: 275-80.
76. Caudana R, Morana G, Pirovano GP, Nicoli N, Portuese A, Spinazzi A, Di Rito R, *et al*. Focal malignant hepatic lesions: MR imaging enhanced with gadolinium benzyloxypropionictetra-acetate (BOPTA)--preliminary results of phase II clinical application. *Radiology* 1996; 199: 513-20.
77. Kreft B, Block W, Dombrowski F, Fackeldey A, Bachmann R, Muhlhauser J, Traber F, *et al*. Diagnostic value of a superparamagnetic iron oxide in MR imaging of chronic liver disease in an animal model. *AJR Am J Roentgenol* 1998; 170: 661-8.
78. Nagata Y, Yamamoto K, Hiraoka M, Abe M, Takahashi M, Akuta K, Nishimura Y, *et al*. Monitoring liver tumor therapy with [18F]FDG positron emission tomography. *J Comput Assist Tomogr* 1990; 14: 370-4.
79. Okazumi S, Isono K, Enomoto K, Kikuchi T, Ozaki M, Yamamoto H, Hayashi H, *et al*. Evaluation of liver tumors using fluorine-18-fluorodeoxyglucose PET: characterization of tumor and assessment of effect of treatment. *J Nucl Med* 1992; 33: 333-9.
80. Khan MA, Combs CS, Brunt EM, Lowe VJ, Wolverson MK, Solomon H, Collins BT, *et al*. Positron emission tomography scanning in the evaluation of hepatocellular carcinoma. *J Hepatol* 2000; 32: 792-7.

81. Schroder O, Trojan J, Zeuzem S, Baum RP. Limited value of fluorine-18-fluorodeoxyglucose PET for the differential diagnosis of focal liver lesions in patients with chronic hepatitis C virus infection. *Nuklearmedizin* 1998; 37: 279-85.
82. Cottone M, Turri M, Caltagirone M, Parisi P, Orlando A, Fiorentino G, Virdone R, *et al*. Screening for hepatocellular carcinoma in patients with Child's A cirrhosis: an 8-year prospective study by ultrasound and alphafetoprotein. *J Hepatol* 1994; 21: 1029-34.
83. Sato Y, Nakata K, Kato Y, Shima M, Ishii N, Koji T, Taketa K, *et al*. Early recognition of hepatocellular carcinoma based on altered profiles of alpha-fetoprotein. *N Engl J Med* 1993; 328: 1802-6.
84. Collier J, Sherman M. Screening for hepatocellular carcinoma. *Hepatology* 1998; 27: 273-8.
85. Kang JY, Lee TP, Yap I, Lun KC. Analysis of cost-effectiveness of different strategies for hepatocellular carcinoma screening in hepatitis B virus carriers. *J Gastroenterol Hepatol* 1992; 7: 463-8.
86. Mima S, Sekiya C, Kanagawa H, Kohyama H, Gotoh K, Mizuo H, Ijiri M, *et al*. Mass screening for hepatocellular carcinoma: experience in Hokkaido, Japan. *J Gastroenterol Hepatol* 1994; 9: 361-5.
87. Sarasin FP, Giostra E, Hadengue A. Cost-effectiveness of screening for detection of small hepatocellular carcinoma in western patients with Child-Pugh class A cirrhosis. *Am J Med* 1996; 101: 422-4.
88. Carter R, Hemingway D, Cooke TG, Pickard R, Poon FW, McKillop JA, McArdle CS. A prospective study of six methods for detection of hepatic colorectal metastases. *Ann R Coll Surg Engl* 1996; 78: 27-30.
89. Yasuhara K, Kimura K, Ohto M, Matsutani S, Ebara M, Tsuchiya Y, Saisho H. Pulsed Doppler in the diagnosis of small liver tumors. *Br J Radiol* 1988; 61: 898-902.
90. Choi BI, Kim TK, Han JK, Chung JW, Park JH, Han MC. Power versus conventional color Doppler sonography: comparison in the depiction of vasculature in liver tumors. *Radiology* 1996; 200: 55-8.
91. Schlief R. Developments in echo-enhancing agents. *Clin Radiol* 1996; 51: 5-7.
92. Harvey CJ, Blomley MJ, Eckersley RJ, Heckemann RA, Butler-Barnes J, Cosgrove DO. Pulse-inversion mode imaging of liver specific microbubbles: improved detection of subcentimetre metastases [letter]. *Lancet* 2000; 355: 807-8.
93. Blomley MJ, Albrecht T, Cosgrove DO, Patel N, Jayaram V, Butler-Barnes J, Eckersley RJ, *et al*. Improved imaging of liver metastases with stimulated acoustic emission in the late phase of enhancement with the US contrast agent SH U 508A: early experience. *Radiology* 1999; 210: 409-16.
94. Sommer G, Olcott EW, Tai L. Liver tumors: utility of characterization at dual-frequency US. *Radiology* 1999; 211: 629-36.
95. Wernecke K, Rummeny E, Bongartz G, Vassallo P, Kivelitz D, Wiesmann W, Peters PE, *et al*. Detection of hepatic masses in patients with carcinoma: comparative sensitivities of sonography, CT, and MR imaging. *AJR Am J Roentgenol* 1991; 157: 731-9.
96. Zeman RK, Fox SH, Silverman PM, Davros WJ, Carter LM, Griego D, Weltman DI, *et al*. Helical (spiral) CT of the abdomen. *AJR Am J Roentgenol* 1993; 160: 719-25.
97. Kuszyk BS, Bluemke DA, Urban BA, Choti MA, Hruban RH, Sitzmann JV, Fishman EK. Portal-phase contrast-enhanced helical CT for the detection of malignant hepatic tumors: sensitivity based on comparison with intraoperative and pathologic findings. *AJR Am J Roentgenol* 1996; 166: 91-5.
98. Oliver JHr, Baron RL, Federle MP, Rockette HE, Jr. Detecting hepatocellular carcinoma: value of unenhanced or arterial phase CT imaging or both used in conjunction with conventional portal venous phase contrast-enhanced CT imaging. *AJR Am J Roentgenol* 1996; 167: 71-7.
99. Oliver JHr, Baron RL, Federle MP, Jones BC, Sheng R. Hypervascular liver metastases: do unenhanced and hepatic arterial phase CT images affect tumor detection? *Radiology* 1997; 205: 709-15.
100. Paulson EK, McDermott VG, Keogan MT, DeLong DM, Frederick MG, Nelson RC. Carcinoid metastases to the liver: role of triple-phase helical CT. *Radiology* 1998; 206: 143-50.
101. Nordlinger B, Guiguet M, Vaillant JC, Balladur P, Boudjema K, Bachellier P, Jaeck D. Surgical resection of colorectal carcinoma metastases to the liver. A prognostic scoring system to improve

case selection, based on 1568 patients. Association Francaise de Chirurgie. *Cancer* 1996; 77: 1254-62.
102. Giacchetti S, Itzhaki M, Gruia G, Adam R, Zidani R, Kunstlinger F, Brienza S, et al. Long-term survival of patients with unresectable colorectal cancer liver metastases following infusional chemotherapy with 5-fluorouracil, leucovorin, oxaliplatin and surgery. *Ann Oncol* 1999; 10: 663-9.
103. Bluemke DA, Fishman EK. Spiral CT arterial portography of the liver. *Radiology* 1993; 186: 576-9.
104. Graf O, Dock WI, Lammer J, Thurnher S, Eibenberger KL, Wildling R, Niederle B, et al. Determination of optimal time window for liver scanning with CT during arterial portography. *Radiology* 1994; 190: 43-7.
105. Young N, Sing T, Wong KP, Hollands M, Tait N. Use of spiral and non-spiral computed tomography arterial portography in the detection of potentially malignant liver masses. *J Gastroenterol Hepatol* 1997; 12: 385-91.
106. Ward J, Naik KS, Guthrie JA, Wilson D, Robinson PJ. Hepatic lesion detection: comparison of MR imaging after the administration of superparamagnetic iron oxide with dual-phase CT by using alternative-free response receiver operating characteristic analysis. *Radiology* 1999; 210: 459-66.
107. Soyer P, Bluemke DA, Hruban RH, Sitzmann JV, Fishman EK. Hepatic metastases from colorectal cancer: detection and false-positive findings with helical CT during arterial portography. *Radiology* 1994; 193: 71-4.
108. Freeny PC, Nghiem HV, Winter TC. Helical CT during arterial portography: optimization of contrast enhancement and scanning parameters. *Radiology* 1995; 194: 83-90.
109. De Lange EE, Mugler JPr, Gay SB, DeAngelis GA, Berr SS, Harris EK. Focal liver disease: comparison of breath-hold T1-weighted MP-GRE MR imaging and contrast-enhanced CT--lesion detection, localization, and characterization. *Radiology* 1996; 200: 465-73.
110. Gaa J, Hatabu H, Jenkins RL, Finn JP, Edelman RR. Liver masses: replacement of conventional T2-weighted spin-echo MR imaging with breath-hold MR imaging. *Radiology* 1996; 200: 459-64.
111. Semelka RC, Schlund JF, Molina PL, Willms AB, Kahlenberg M, Mauro MA, Weeks SM, et al. Malignant liver lesions: comparison of spiral CT arterial portography and MR imaging for diagnostic accuracy, cost, and effect on patient management. *J Magn Reson Imaging* 1996; 6: 39-43.
112. Semelka RC, Cance WG, Marcos HB, Mauro MA. Liver metastases: comparison of current MR techniques and spiral CT during arterial portography for detection in 20 surgically staged cases. *Radiology* 1999; 213: 86-91.
113. Lencioni R, Donati F, Cioni D, Paolicchi A, Cicorelli A, Bartolozzi C. Detection of colorectal liver metastases: prospective comparison of unenhanced and ferumoxides-enhanced magnetic resonance imaging at 1.5 T, dual-phase spiral CT, and spiral CT during arterial portography. *MAGMA* 1998; 7: 76-87.
114. Hagspiel KD, Neidl KF, Eichenberger AC, Weder W, Marincek B. Detection of liver metastases: comparison of superparamagnetic iron oxide-enhanced and unenhanced MR imaging at 1.5 T with dynamic CT, intraoperative US, and percutaneous US. *Radiology* 1995; 196: 471-8.
115. Paul MA, Mulder LS, Cuesta MA, Sikkenk AC, Lyesen GK, Meijer S. Impact of intraoperative ultrasonography on treatment strategy for colorectal cancer. *Br J Surg* 1994; 81: 1660-3.
116. Soyer P, Levesque M, Elias D, Zeitoun G, Roche A. Detection of liver metastases from colorectal cancer: comparison of intraoperative US and CT during arterial portography. *Radiology* 1992; 183: 541-4.
117. Bilchik AJ, Wood TF, Allegra D, Tsioulias GJ, Chung M, Rose DM, Ramming KP, et al. Cryosurgical ablation and radiofrequency ablation for unresectable hepatic malignant neoplasms: a proposed algorithm. *Arch Surg* 2000; 135: 657-62.
118. Feld RI, Liu JB, Nazarian L, Lev-Toaff AS, Needleman L, Rawool NM, Merton DA, et al. Laparoscopic liver sonography: preliminary experience in liver metastases compared with CT portography. *J Ultrasound Med* 1996; 15: 288-95.

119. Barbot DJ, Marks JH, Feld RI, Liu JB, Rosato FE. Improved staging of liver tumors using laparoscopic intraoperative ultrasound. *J Surg Oncol* 1997; 64: 63-7.
120. Lebtahi R, Cadiot G, Sarda L, Daou D, Faraggi M, Petegnief Y, Mignon M, *et al*. Clinical impact of somatostatin receptor scintigraphy in the management of patients with neuroendocrine gastroenteropancreatic tumors. *J Nucl Med* 1997; 38: 853-8.
121. Frilling A, Malago M, Martin H, Broelsch CE. Use of somatostatin receptor scintigraphy to image extrahepatic metastases of neuroendocrine tumors. *Surgery* 1998; 124: 1000-4.
122. Chiti A, Fanti S, Savelli G, Romeo A, Bellanova B, Rodari M, van Graafeiland BJ, *et al*. Comparison of somatostatin receptor imaging, computed tomography and ultrasound in the clinical management of neuroendocrine gastro-entero-pancreatic tumors. *Eur J Nucl Med* 1998; 25: 1396-403.
123. Nazarian LN, Park JH, Halpern EJ, Parker L, Johnson PT, Lev-Toaff AS, Wechsler RJ. Size of colorectal liver metastases at abdominal CT: comparison of precontrast and postcontrast studies. *Radiology* 1999; 213: 825-30.
124. Hustinx R, Paulus P, Jacquet N, Jerusalem G, Bury T, Rigo P. Clinical evaluation of whole-body 18F-fluorodeoxyglucose positron emission tomography in the detection of liver metastases. *Ann Oncol* 1998; 9: 397-401.
125. Warren HW, Gallagher H, Hemingway DM, Angerson WJ, Bessent RG, Wotherspoon H, McArdle CS, *et al*. Prospective assessment of the hepatic perfusion index in patients with colorectal cancer. *Br J Surg* 1998; 85: 1708-12.
126. De Santis M, Cristani A, Cioni G, Casolo A, Canossi G, Ventura E, Romagnoli R. The magnetic resonance of small hepatocarcinoma. A comparison with echography, computed tomography, digital angiography and computed tomography with lipiodol. *Radiol Med (Torino)* 1992; 84: 587-95.
127. Ueda K, Kitagawa K, Kadoya M, Matsui O, Takashima T, Yamahana T. Detection of hypervascular hepatocellular carcinoma by using spiral volumetric CT: comparison of US and MR imaging. *Abdom Imaging* 1995; 20: 547-53.
128. Bartolozzi C, Lencioni R, Caramella D, Palla A, Bassi AM, Di Candio G. Small hepatocellular carcinoma. Detection with US, CT, MR imaging, DSA, and Lipiodol-CT. *Acta Radiol* 1996; 37: 69-74.
129. Schneider F, Chapuis L, Gillet M, Leyvraz S, Schnyder P, Meuli R. Détection des lésions focales hépatiques malignes. Comparaison de l'échographie, de la porto-tomodensitométrie, de la tomodensitométrie tardive et de l'imagerie par résonance magnétique. *Gastroenterol Clin Biol* 1999; 23: 105-13.

CT imaging of colonic tumors: hydro-CT and virtual colonoscopy

Pierre-Jean Valette[1], Jean-Christophe Saurin[2], Pascale Fouque[1], Denis Marion[2]

[1] Département des Spécialités Digestives, Hôpital Édouard-Herriot, Lyon, France
[2] Service de Radiologie, Hôtel-Dieu, Lyon, France

CT of the abdomen and pelvis was initially considered for solid organs only, and the bowel was simply labelled with oral or rectal contrast so that it could be easily identified and distinguished from any disease. In such conditions the CT imaging of the bowel wall was limited to the incidental visualization of large tumors. Recently the spiral technology has opened new fields of clinical applications of CT, most of them focused on the investigation of bowel diseases. For instance, the major role that CT can play in cases of acute abdomen is now well-documented and CT is widely used in emergency cases. The use of CT for the detection of the bowel tumors is more recent and still under evaluation. We will describe in this paper the various techniques of large bowel CT imaging including the virtual colonoscopy. We will also present a review of the published data for the diagnosis of the colonic tumors.

Technical background

Spiral CT enables the examination of the entire abdomen with thin slices in one rapid sequence. There are several advantages with this technology. As the study can be completed in a single breath-hold, misregistration artefacts caused by uneven inspiration are eliminated. The reduced scanning means also that, when intravenous iodine contrast enhancement is needed, the entire part of the body that is being studied can be imaged at a peak contrast. Most importantly, data acquisition during spiral CT is continuous and therefore volumetric. Although images are initially presented as single axial slices for convenience, cinedisplay, any other 2D planar reformatting, and 3D pictures are then available from a truly three dimensional dataset.

Technique of exploration

The CT protocol consists of an helical acquisition through the entire colon with overlapping thin slices of 2 or 3 mm. The acquisition is obtained during a single 30-45 seconds breath-hold, depending on the length of exploration. For a visualisation in exquisite details the bowel wall needs to fulfil the following criteria: full bowel preparation, significant distension of the lumen, adequate tissue contrast, and temporary paralysis. Colon preparation is similar to the one performed before a real colonoscopy. Colon paralysis is obtained by IV smooth muscle relaxant administration. Distension and adequate bowel wall contrast may be obtained in two different ways:

- **The colon lumen may be filled with 2 L of water**. Once satisfactory distension has been achieved, spiral CT is performed to encompass the entire colon 50 seconds after an IV injection of 120 to 150 ml of contrast medium. This technique, often named "hydro-CT" in the literature, has also been applied to the small bowel for tumor detection after a water enteroclysis. It is interesting to notice that the possibility of exploring the bowel by CT with a clear depiction of stenosing lesions has been first recognized in cases of obstruction in which a spontaneous fluid distension of the lumen is present [1]. Once the slices have been obtained, they can be simply visualized in a cinedisplay mode which offers an efficient way to follow the bowel loops. Multiplanar reconstructions may also be performed in order to obtain cuts along the longitudinal axis of the bowel. It has been shown that a better analysis of strictured bowel could be achieved in such a way.

- **The colon lumen may be distended by air insufflation**. Since the density of air is significantly lower than the colon wall's, there is no need for IV contrast injection. The study is generally repeated with the patient lying supine and prone to ensure that all colonic segments have been imaged distended and free of remaining fluid. After acquisition, the data are downloaded to an independent workstation equipped with appropriate software for rendering perspective and volume. The considerable difference in image contrast between the intraluminal gas and the colon wall makes this interface an easy target for the rendering of 3D pictures, allowing creation of a graphical representation of the colon that simulates an endoscopic view. The "virtual colonoscopy" may then be performed by the use of "fly through" navigation tools simulating the progression of an endoscope within the colon. Image analysis is interactive, and the radiologist can choose to move within the antegrade and retrograde colon, to view the rendering mucosa from any angle and to pass through strictures.

It is important here to notice a major difference between the hydro-CT technique and the virtual colonoscopy. With hydro-CT the picture is not limited to the bowel surface and the colon lumen as well as the wall and the pericolic spaces can be analysed at the same time. Contrast uptake of colon wall thickening may also be analysed for better identification of the lesions, and adequate cleansing of the lumen is not so critical as it is for a virtual colonoscopy. In the literature, hydro-CT has mainly been studied for the diagnosis and local spread of large colonic tumors. With virtual colonoscopy, although the primary transverse slices analysis is always possible, the study is focused on the mucosal surface deformations due to protruding lesions. The main reported application is the detection of polyps.

Normal results and semiology of the colonic tumors

On cut slices, the colonic wall appears after distension as a regular well-defined hyperdense line 2 to 3 mm thick. Conversely to high resolution US, the parietal layers are not visible, except for some cases of colitis. The colon diameter varies from 5 to 10 cm. The colonic surface is regular and, in virtual colonoscopy, the haustrations may hide small tumors as they do in real colonoscopy.

In patients with colorectal cancer, hydro-CT typically demonstrates a discrete soft-tissue mass or a local thickening of the wall. The sharpness of tumor edges with the adjacent normal colon usually allows easy distinction from inflammatory lesions. The tumor enhancement by the IV contrast injection is variable. The tumor may narrow the colonic lumen with fluid distension above in case of obstruction. The deepest part of the tumor may also be analysed for diagnosis of local spread to the pericolic fat *(figure 1)* or neighbouring organs [2]. When enlarged, the lymph nodes are visualized as rounded structures adjacent to the tumor or more distant, within the mesosigmoid or the retroperitoneum. On virtual colonoscopy, tumors are visualized as parietal lesions more or less protruding inside the lumen. A pedunculated polyp is identified by means of its stalk *(figure 2)*, whereas a sessile polyp appears as a polypoid soft-tissue mass projecting into the air-filled lumen of the colon. However, flat adenomas (lesions raised less than 2 mm from the surface of the colon) are difficult to detect. In case of colorectal cancer, the intraluminal disease and the presence of a stricture can be evaluated. The extraluminal part of the tumor may also be analysed on the transverse axial cuts. Pseudolesions that can produce false-positive findings at virtual colonoscopy include the ileocecal valve, retained stool, retained barium, respiratory artifacts, and a stool-filled diverticulum. Most of these pitfalls, however, can be avoided be a systematic comparison of 2D and 3D pictures [3].

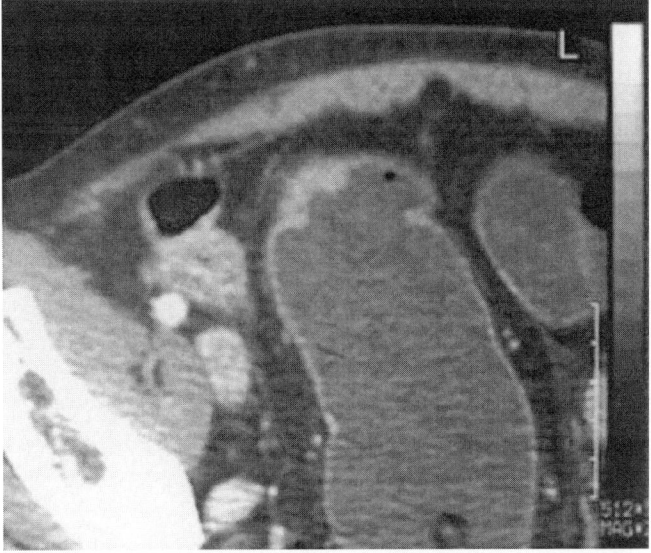

Figure 1. Hydro-CT: small ulcerated cancer of the recto-sigmoid. There is evidence of fat stranding of the deep part of the tumor consistant with a local extension (T3).

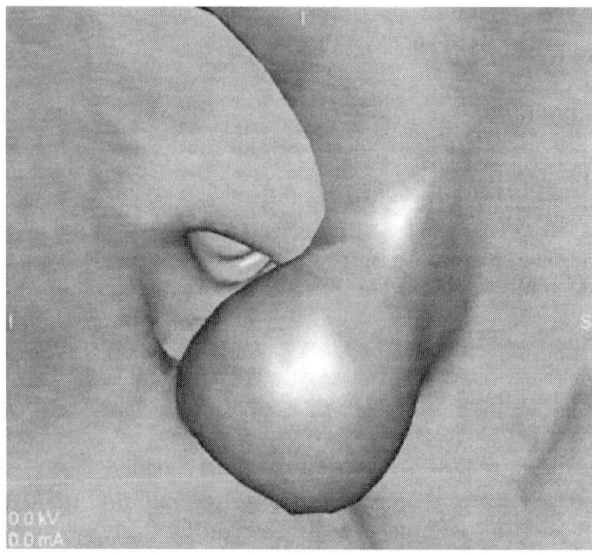

Figure 2. Virtual colonoscopy : 12 mm pedonculated polyp hanging into the left colon lumen.

Results

Cancer diagnosis

Although hydro-CT is a simple procedure with no need for a complex post-processing, very few studies have been published about this technique. One feasibility study [4] reporting 35 cases of patients with proven colonic cancer has been published in 1992. The CT, performed without information from the colonoscopy, was able to detect the tumor in all cases. Tumor location at hydro-CT was always well correlated with the surgical findings. Virtual colonoscopy allows similar results. Two series focused on the diagnosis of cancer [5, 6] showed that all tumors over 2 cm could be evidenced by virtual colonoscopy. All these results however bring no information about the accuracy of hydro-CT or virtual colonoscopy for cancer screening since all included patients had a tumor. The series published by Lipscomb [7] in 1996 is, for this reason, of specific interest. This prospective work concerns 72 elderly patients examined because of colonic symptoms, and thus justifying colonic investigations to rule out the presence of a cancer. The result of CT was in agreement with that of colonoscopy in 70% of cases, and all 6 cancers proven at endoscopy were prospectively detected.

CT has also been proposed for investigation of patients with incomplete colonoscopic exploration. Fenlon [8] prospectively examined 29 patients with a colonic tumoral stricture preventing the colonoscopic study of the colon above the tumor. All 29 cancers could be evidenced by virtual colonoscopy. Two cancers and 24 polyps close to the tumor could also be identified. All these synchronous lesions, except one polyp, were confirmed at surgery or postoperative colonoscopy. Only 2 polyps were missed.

Polyps screening

Ten studies reporting the results of virtual colonoscopy for the diagnosis of colonic polyps have been published until now [9-18]. All these studies were prospective, the CT being performed just before the real colonoscopy and analysed without knowing its result. The colonoscopy was always the gold standard. The results are reported in terms of sensitivity and specificity, for the detection of each polyp, or for the detection of patients with polyps. The number of included patients varied from 10 to 180. Complete results are summarized in *table I*.

Table I. Sensitivity and specificity of virtual colonoscopy for polyps screening.

Reference	N° of pts	N° of pts with polyps	N° of polyps	Sensivity (by polyps)	%	Sensitivity (by patients)	%	Specificity (by patients)	%
Hara 1996 [9]	10	9	18	All > 10 mm = 5-9 mm < 5 mm	40-50 100 71 11-28	> 10 mm = 5-9 mm < 5 mm	100 71 29-43		
Hara 1997 [3]	70		115	> 10 mm = 5-9 mm < 5 mm	67-73 56-69 25-27	> 10 mm = 5-9 mm < 5 mm	75-75 68-64 43-40	> 10 mm = 5-9 mm < 5 mm	90-91 58-67 75-85
Fenlon 1999 [11]	100	49	115	All > 10 mm = 5-9 mm < 5 mm	71 91 82 55	All > 10 mm = 5-9 mm	82 96 92	All > 10 mm = 5-9 mm	84 96 94
Rex 1999 [13]	46	33	91	All > 10 mm = 5-9 mm < 5 mm	22 60 43 11	> 10 mm = 5-9 mm < 5 mm	83 43 25		
Kay 2000 [12]	38		24	> 10 mm = 5-9 mm < 5 mm	91 62 38	> 10 mm = 5-9 mm	90 66	> 10 mm = 5-9 mm	82 75
Naus 1997 [14]	25					> 5 mm < 5 mm	100 43	> 5 mm < 5 mm	82 78
Pineau 1999 [16]	88	33	86			All > 10 mm = 5-9 mm	72 100 94	All > 10 mm = 5-9 mm	61 87 70
Bethge 1999 [15]	22		55	All > 10 mm = 5-9 mm < 5 mm	33 100 65 15	All	21	All	25
Fletcher 1999 [17]	180		420			> 10 mm > 5 mm	85 88	All (?)	93
Geetanjali 1999 [18]	119	44	181			All	88	All	64

The result of the analysis of these published data is that the average sensitivity of the virtual colonoscopy for the diagnosis of polyps over 10 mm is 80% when analysed by polyps, and 85% when analysed by patients. The average specificity is 83%. The sensitivity falls to 62% for polyps between 5 and 10 mm, and 27% under 5 mm. The wide range of the results is however noticeable, with a sensitivity varying from 21% to 88% and a specificity from 25% to 84% (including all sizes of polyps and patient basis analysis). There are several reasons for these variations. The virtual colonoscopy is a recent and still evolving technique. Differences in material and software performances may be advanced, as well as the investigators' unequal skill. Regarding sensitivity, all false negative cases concerning polyps larger than 5 mm have been retrospectively reviewed in the 4 largest series [10-13]. Almost 50% of the missed polyps could be definitively identified. In the other cases, the suboptimal preparation and the insufficient distension of some parts of the colon were advocated. Only one publication [11] focused on the retrospective evaluation of polyps smaller than 5 mm. The conclusion was that most of them could not be clearly evidenced, even with optimal conditions. Flat polyps also appear to be a limitation to the CT detection as such lesions have never been evidenced on these studies. These data suggest that the detection of polyps thicker than 5 mm might be improved, or at least might become more reproducible, with a better proficiency of the investigators and technical improvement. The multidetector array technology CT, which allows a faster image acquisition with thinner slices, and the possible automated software detection of the polyps will also probably improve the results in the future.

Examination tolerance and complications

The virtual colonoscopy is a non-invasive technique, needs no anaesthesia and, until now, has no reported complication. The X-ray exposition is similar to the one provided with a double contrast enema and therefore is acceptable. However the virtual colonoscopy has some constraints since the bowel cleansing should be as complete as it is for a real colonoscopy and because the amount of inflated air is dictated by the threshold of pain. In such conditions it might be considered less comfortable than an exploration performed under general anaesthesia. No study has been performed at the present time to assess the tolerance of this examination.

Clinical applications

Cancer diagnosis

The limited data about the diagnosis of colonic cancer by hydro-CT or virtual colonoscopy do not authorize any recommandation about the use of these techniques in replacement of a conventional colonoscopy for patients with clinical suspicion of cancer. However there is evidence that hydro-CT allows a clear depiction of most cancers, even without bowel preparation. It is therefore possible to suggest the use of hydro-CT in some selected clinical situations :

– when a cancer has been proven by endoscopy and biopsies, a preoperative abdominal CT is often demanded for general evaluation and hepatic metastases screening. If performed on the same occasion, the hydro-CT would not generate additional constraint for the patient, nor extra costs, and it could provide useful informations on the tumor location and local spread. It has been shown [19-21] that 15% to 20% of the colorectal cancers were incorrectly localized by colonoscopy inducing a modified surgical strategy in 8% of cases. The CT could also occasionally evidence proximal tumors in case of incomplete colonoscopy;

– in case of bowel obstruction due to a tumor, the proximal colon is generally spontaneously distended with fluid. A simple water enema of the distal colon combined with thin slices on the strictured zone produces conditions of examination similar to those obtained with the hydro-CT technique. The diagnosis of tumor obstruction becomes then obvious and definite informations on the tumor site can be obtained before an emergency surgery;

– elderly patients with increased risk of colonoscopy and/or anaesthesia complications form the third possible indication of hydro-CT for cancer screening. Although this suggestion is based on the results of a single paper, it appears that the colonoscopists themselves often prefer a non-invasive and low risk technique for evaluation of such patients, the colonoscopy beeing performed consecutively only in case of serious suspicion of tumor. The barium enema which is often requested in such a situation could be efficiently replaced by a water-CT, which is easier to perform and is better tolerated by patients.

The interest of such a use of the hydro-CT still has to be evaluated in prospective studies.

Polyp screening

The choice of a screening method is subject to definite prerequisites: proven accuracy (sensitivity, specificity, PPV, NPV) for the detection of the disease, lack of adverse effects and complications, good patient tolerance, and acceptable costs on a large basis use. There is evidence that, at the present time, none of these criteria except the lack of complication is fulfilled by the virtual colonoscopy. All the published series are limited as regards the number of patients. Although encouraging, the results present major variations raising the question of the reproducibility of the method, and no serious evaluation of the interobserver variability has been published. Even more important is the frequent bias of selection of the studied cases. The reported series include patients who generally run a risk of tumor due to a familial history of colorectal neoplasia, or a rectal bleeding and/or positive fecal blood-test. The prevalence of colorectal neoplasia is therefore high and the results may not be extrapolated to a non-selected population as it would be in a mass screening purpose. Another limitation is the choice of the real colonoscopy for gold standard. Several recent studies [22, 23] comparing a colonoscopy to a second one performed by another investigator or to a surgical exploration have shown that up to 25% of adenomatous polyps and 5% of cancers (2,8% of advanced cancers) could be missed. The reasons for these false negatives are, in most of cases, an incomplete evaluation due to difficult technical conditions. It is therefore difficult to determine what could be the role of the virtual colonoscopy in the colorectal neoplasia screening strategies. The answer will certainly be conditioned by the clinical context and differ for patients with high or low risk of tumor.

Another question is the place of the virtual colonoscopy in relation with the fecal blood test. There is no paper comparing the efficacy of the CT technique and the fecal test for colorectal neoplasia screening. Moreover, CT may not be proposed as a primary test for economic reasons. On the other hand, the fecal test appears to have a good specificity ranging from 90% to 98% but a low positive predictive value ranging from 10% to 17% [24]. This means that 6 to 10 asymptomatic patients with a positive test should be submitted to a colonoscopy to diagnose one cancer. Since complications of the real colonoscopy may be observed with a risk from 0.06% to 0.1% of perforation or bleeding, and 0.01% to 0.03% of mortality, the need for a non-invasive exploration in patients with positive fecal test but a low risk of cancer may be raised. If, for such patients, a sensitivity around 80-90% for the detection of polyps over 10 mm appears to be acceptable, the virtual colonoscopy might become a valuable alternate method to the conventional colonoscopy. The final answer will probably need further prospective studies comparing the effect of these different strategies on the decrease of colorectal cancers, as it has already been demonstrated for the conventional colonoscopy.

Conclusion

Virtual colonoscopy is in the early stages of its development. Its feasibility is now clearly demonstrated, and larger multicentre studies are needed to determine its sensitivity and specificity with reproducible results. The recently introduced multi-slice spiral CT technology, the future refinement in the volume rendering techniques and software automatic detection of lesions, and also the methods of tagging of the fecal residue in order to avoid the bowel cleansing, will also have to be evaluated. Finally, the role of these CT techniques will have to be determined with regard to their potential as a screening tool, their performance in a large population, their cost, patient acceptability and availability.

References

1. Frager D, Rovno HD, Baer JW, Bashist B, Friedman M. Prospective evaluation of colonic obstruction with computed tomography. *Abdom Imaging* 1998; 23 (2): 141-6.
2. Farouk R, Nelson H, Radice E, Mercill S, Gunderson L. Accuracy of computed tomography in determining resectability for locally advanced primary or recurrent colorectal cancers. *Am J Surg* 1998; 175 (4): 283-7.
3. Hara A, Daniel Johnson C, Reed J. Colorectal lesions: evaluation with CT colography. *Radiographics* 1997; 17: 1157-67.
4. Gossios KJ, Tsianos EV, Kontogiannis DS, Demou LL, Tatsis CK, Papakostas VP, Merkouropoulos MM, Tsimoyiannis EC. Water as contrast medium for computed tomography study of colonic wall lesions. *Gastrointest Radiol* 1992; 17 (2): 125-8.
5. Fenlon HM, McAneny DB, Nunes DP, Clarke PD, Ferrucci JT. Occlusive colon carcinoma: virtual colonoscopy in the preoperative evaluation of the proximal colon. *Radiology* 1999; 210 (2): 423-8.
6. Royster AP, Fenlon HM, Clarke PD, Nunes DP, Ferrucci JT. CT colonoscopy of colorectal neoplasms: two-dimensional and three-dimensional virtual-reality techniques with colonoscopic correlation. *AJR Am J Roentgenol* 1997; 169 (5): 1237-42.

7. Lipscomb G, Loughrey G, Thakker M, Rees W, Nicholson D. A prospective study of abdominal computerized tomography and colonoscopy in the diagnosis of colonic disease in an elderly population. *Eur J Gastroenterol Hepatol* 1996; 8 (9): 887-91.
8. Fenlon HM. Colorectal neoplasm detection using virtual colonoscopy: a feasibility study. *Gastrointest Endosc* 2000; 51 (3): 369-71.
9. Hara A, Daniel Johnson C, Reed J, *et al*. Detection of colorectal polyps by CT colography: feasibility of a novel technique. *Gastroenterology* 1996; 110: 284-90.
10. Hara A, Daniel Johnson C, Reed J, *et al*. Detection of colorectal polyps with CT colography: initial assessment of sensitivity and specificity. *Radiology* 1997; 205: 59-65.
11. Fenlon HM, Nunes DP, Schroy PC 3rd, Barish MA, Clarke PD, Ferrucci JT. A comparison of virtual and conventional colonoscopy for the detection of colorectal polyps. *N Engl J Med* 1999; 341 (20): 1496-503.
12. Kay CL, Kulling D, Hawes RH, Young JW, Cotton PB. Virtual endoscopy comparison with colonoscopy in the dectection of space occupying lesions of the colon. *Endoscopy* 2000; 32 (3): 226-32.
13. Rex DK, Vining D, Kopecky KK. An initial experience with screening for colon polyps using spiral CT with and without CT colography. *Gastrointest Endosc* 1999; 50 (3): 309-13.
14. Naus M. Prospective comparisons of virtual colonoscopy in the detection of polyps. *Gastrointest Endosc* 1997; 45 : AB113.
15. Bethge N, Breitkreutz C, Rothsteil R, Baron J. Prospective controlled double-blinded trial of virtual colonoscopy in occult GI bleeding. *Am J Gastroenterol* 1999; 116: A378.
16. Pineau B, Mikulaninec C, Vining D. Ability of virtual colonoscopy to detect patients with colorectal polyps. *Gastroenterology* 1999; 116: A485.
17. Fletcher J. CT colonography in 180 patients: the benefits of prone imaging. *Gastroenterology* 1999; 116: A404.
18. Geetanjali A. Sensitivity and specificity of virtual colonoscopy for detection of colorectal neoplasia. *Gastroenterology* 1999; 116: A44.
19. Vignati P, Welch JP, Cohen JL. Endoscopic localization of colon cancers. *Surg Endosc* 1994; 8: 1085-7.
20. Hancock JH, Talbot RW. Accuracy of colonoscopy in localisation of colorectal cancer. *Int J Colorectal Dis* 1995; 10: 140-1.
21. Lam DT, Kwong KH, Lam CW, Leong HT, Kwok SP. How useful is colonoscopy in locating colorectal lesions. *Surg Endosc* 1998; 12: 839-41.
22. Gorski TF, Rosen L, Riether R, Stasik J, Khubchandani I. Colorectal cancer after surveillance colonoscopy: false-negative examination or fast growth? *Dis Colon Rectum* 1999; 42: 877-80.
23. Rex DK, Cutler CS, Lemmel GT, Rahmani Ey, Clark DW, Helper DJ. Colonoscopics miss rates of adenomas determined by back-to-back colonoscopies. *Gastroenterology* 1997; 112: 24-8.
24. Winaver SJ, Fletcher RH, Miller L, Godlee F, Stolar MH, Mulrow CD. Colorectal cancer screening : clinical guidelines and rationale. *Gastroenterology* 1997; 112: 594-642.

Laparoscopy: revival of an old technique?

Axel Eickhoff, Arne R.J. Schneider, Joachim C. Arnold, Jürgen F. Riemann

Medical Department C, Klinikum Ludwigshafen, Ludwigshafen, Germany

Laparoscopy was introduced into the gastroenterologists armamentarium in a time when rigid endoscopic devices, *e.g.* the rigid gastroscope, were used regularly. It is therefore one of the oldest endoscopic methods and was firstly described by Kelling in 1902 [1]. Other pioneers in this field like Kalk initiated the spread of this method and introduced the term laparoscopy [2]. Diagnostic laparoscopy was described as a routine method especially for the diagnosis of liver diseases and tumor staging. Newer imaging techniques like CT-scan, ultrasonography (US), magnetic resonance imaging (MRI) and recently endoscopic ultrasonography (EUS) seemed to be more accurate in evaluating abdominal disorders; this led to a steadily decline of laparoscopy in the 1970's and 1980's.

This was the time period when surgical colleagues embraced and expanded laparoscopy technique more and more for therapeutic indications. Today therapeutic laparoscopy has been established in the armamentarium of surgeons and gynecologists worldwide. Based on the decline of diagnostic laparoscopy by gastroenterologists, even in the departments of its biggest advocacy, more and more surgeons discover the potential benefit of laparoscopy in the diagnostic approach either. One reason is the fact that appropriate education and training programs are lacking for gastroenterologists [3].

In the 1990's there have been a "new" interest and a remarkable revitalization in diagnostic laparoscopy, expressed by a number of publications [3-5]. This was based on prospective comparative studies which revealed crucial limitations of the new imaging techniques (US, CT), especially in depicting early liver metastasis and peritoneal tumor spread. New treatment options in viral hepatitis and chronic liver disease ask for a more accurate diagnostic work-up. The high miss rate of percutaneous liver biopsy for the detection of cirrhosis has repeatedly been reported; on the other hand there is emerging evidence of the high accuracy of laparoscopy and direct vision biopsy [6].

Today, on the step to the next millenium, the renewed interest in this "old" technique is based on additional introduction of small diameter laparoscopes, laparoscopic ultrasonography and further immunological staining methods. Laparoscopy is an invasive diagnostic tool with comparable or superior results to other imaging modalities, it is a safe and cost-effective diagnostic method for various gastrointestinal disorders *(table I)*.

Table I. Present indications for diagnostic laparoscopy.

- Staging of GI-malignancies
- Chronic liver disease
- Focal liver disease
- Ascites of unknown cause
  (Acute abdomen, blunt / penetrating abdominal trauma)

Technique

Based on the above-mentioned history of laparoscopy, different laparoscopy techniques emerged on the site of the gastroenterologists on the one hand and on the surgery site on the other. Gastroenterologists perform laparoscopy usually as a single diagnostic procedure in the endoscopy unit using only sedation and analgesia. Surgeons embedded laparoscopy usually in their therapeutic approach performing laparoscopy in the operating room under general anesthesia immediately before laparotomy.

For diagnostic laparoscopy by gastroenterologists premedication under permanently controlled pulseoxymetry consists of a tranquilizer (*e.g.* midazolam 3-10 mg) and an opiate (*e.g.* pethidine 50-100 mg). The pneumoperitoneum is achieved by insertion of the Veres needle at the point of Monroe and insufflation of nitrous oxide up to an intraperitoneal pressure of 12-15 mmHg. For insertion of the main trocar, usually the left paramedian approach (point of Kalk) is used. Various diameter laparoscopes are used to examine the abdominal cavity. In our institution the following inspection schema is used: intraabdominal localization of the Veres needle, left and right lobes of the liver with the ligamentum teres, gallbladder, stomach, spleen, omentum, peritoneal wall and the visible parts of the colon and the small bowel. A second puncture using 2-3.5 mm trocars is used for the needle biopsy. This approach offers the advantage of achieving hemostasis after liver biopsies either by direct pressure *via* a palpation probe or a coagulation probe. For liver biopsies various needle types are available (*e.g.* Menghini, Silverman, Tru-cut). Suspicious lesions suggesting metastases or primary hepatic tumors are biopsied by using forceps.

The availability of small diameter laparoscopes has been a recent development in instrumentation [7]. This technique requires only one trocar for both the insertion of the Veres needle and the 1.9 mm optic. Small diameter laparoscopes offer certain advantages as a consequence of their minimal invasiveness. It has been shown that diagnostic laparoscopy with this new technique could be performed as safely in high risk patients with an INR > 2 and/ or a platelet count of < 50/ nl, other coagulopathies or massive portal hypertension. Disadvantages include limited oblique vision due to the prograde optic and the limited lucidity.

Staging of gastrointestinal malignancies

The most important reason for performing staging laparoscopy in patients with solid malignant abdominal tumors is the avoidance of unnecessary surgery. Multiple studies have repeatedly demonstrated that laparoscopy is superior to other imaging techniques (CT, US) even in the face of the latest technology. An accurate diagnosis by laparoscopy is achieved in up to 80-90% of all cases [8]. The advantage of laparoscopy over CT and US is the detection of small lesions of just a few millimeters, peritoneal metastases or focal lesions directly on the surface of the liver with the possibility of an immediate biopsy.

Prospective studies presented the high rate of false-negative results of CT-scans in depicting small metastatic lesions. In three prospective studies, laparoscopy detected previously unsuspected metastatic lesions in up to 48% of cases stressing the diagnostic yield of this method [9-11]. The negative predictive value for CT-scan was only 50% compared to 89% for laparoscopy.

In a retrospective trial from our department, metastases were detected in 21 in 89 patients (23.6%) with diagnostic laparoscopy prior to intended curative resection. Due to the laparoscopically detected metastases, laparotomies in curative intention were avoided in 9/49 patients (18.4%) with gastric cancer, 11/33 patients (33%) with pancreatic cancer and one patient with adenocarcinoma of the esophagus. Referring to the avoidance of laparotomies, various authors demonstrated similar results *(table II)*. The diagnostic yield can be increased by brush cytology or cytological staining of peritoneal washings [12]. In search of higher diagnostic accuracy for the detection of intraabdominal metastases, light-induced fluorescence methods (LIFD) were adapted to laparoscopy. Consequently in up to 17.5% laparoscopy with LIFD increased the detection of tumors by 17.5%. Further trials should deal with the question which metastases can be visualized by LIFD and whether the detection of micrometastases of less than 1 mm in diameter is relevant for the prognosis of patients.

Table II. Avoidable laparotomies by staging laparoscopy.

Authors	N° of pts	Primary tumor	Avoidable n =	Laparotomies %
O'Brien et al. [13]	106	Esophagus, stomach	29	27.4
Molloy et al. [14]	244	Esophagus, stomach	92	37.7
Possik et al. [19]	360	Stomach	123	34.2
Conlon et al. [16]	92	Stomach	31	33.7
Warshaw et al. [11]	40	Pancreas	14	35
Fernandez et al. [12]	114	Pancreas	27	23.7
Own data	49	Stomach	9	18.4
Own data	33	Pancreas	11	33.3

The above mentioned high accuracy of laparoscopy in detecting metastases of solid gastrointestinal tumors is well-known; however there is a wide range of sensitivity rates published in the literature [11-20] *(tables III and IV)*.

Table III. Sensitivity and specificity for laparoscopy staging of gastric cancer.

Authors	N° of pts	Sensitivity %	Specificity %
O'Brien et al. [13]	145	77	-
Molloy et al. [14]	244	81.4	-
Possik et al. [19]	360	83.3	100
Watt et al. [17]	90	51-89	97-100
Kriplani et al. [18]	40	87	-
Own data	48	64.3	100

Table IV. Sensitivity and specificity for laparoscopy staging of pancreatic cancer.

Authors	N° of pts	Sensitivity %	Specificity %
Warshaw et al. [11]	40	82.4	98
Fernandez et al. [12]	114	93.1	100
Conlon et al. [16]	108	91	100
Reed et al. [15]	11	22.2	100
Bemelman et al. [20]	70	76	-
Own data	33	73.3	100

Compared with laparoscopy in internal medicine, surgical laparoscopy aims at a complete evaluation of potential metastases also at the crura of the diaphragm, the omental bursa and the perivascular regions. These regions play a crucial role particularly in the staging of distal esophageal, gastric and pancreatic cancer. One major obstacle of the "internistic" laparoscopy is the fact that only the abdominal cavity can be inspected sufficiently, whereas local tumor spread cannot be correctly evaluated. Regarding the resectability, a correct statement of local tumor expansion is particularly important in pancreatic and common bile duct tumors. Further limitations are based on the fact that only 70% of the liver surface is visible at laparoscopy; the diagnostic laparoscopy is not able to depict deep liver metastases and adhesions may not be detectable sufficiently.

Emerging new techniques appear at the horizon trying to improve these weak points of diagnostic laparoscopy. In addition to a thorough work-up of intraabdominal structures, laparoscopic sonography and Doppler ultrasound may increase diagnostic yield by visualisation of minor intrahepatic metastases and direct assessment of local tumor spread. By introducing ultrasound into laparoscopic techniques, surgeons try to fill in the gap between non-invasive imaging techniques (US,CT,MRI) and intraoperative ultrasound. In the paper of Rahusen et al., the latter is considered the most sensitive method for the detection of liver metastases in colorectal carcinoma [21]. Laparoscopy with laparoscopic ultrasound (lapUS) identified metastases in 18 out of 47 patients (38%). Remarkably, only 6 patients were ruled out as candidates for resection solely by laparoscopy whereas further 12 patients with unresectable metastases were recognised by lapUS.

The introduction of additional "mini"-laparoscopy (1,9 mm in diameter) could lead to an improving view of primary invisible parts of the abdomen. Overall, the use of laparoscopy in the diagnostic work-up of gastrointestinal tumors could lead to a more accurate report of the tumor stage. Possible additional information which could be achieved by laparoscopy is crucially dependent on interindividual techniques, the examiner's expertise and the use of lapUS. Laparoscopy and lapUS are particularly valuable for evaluating the resectability of pancreatic and hepatobiliary tumors with regard to local tumor involvement and vessel infiltration.

Chronic liver disease and focal liver disease

Over the years, the diagnosis of liver cirrhosis and its possible endstage of hepatocellular carcinoma remain to be the main indication for laparoscopy and guided biopsy. The diagnosis of cirrhosis is connected with crucial clinical consequences. For example, an interferon therapy is contraindicated in patients with chronic hepatitis B (HBV-) infection and advanced liver cirrhosis. Furthermore, chronic hepatitis C (HCV-) infection and simultaneous cirrhosis lead to a reduced virological and serological response of an interferon therapy to a minimum [22]. Additionally, the new treatment modalities not only for viral hepatitis but also for autoimmunhepatitis, hemochromatosis, Wilson's-disease or primary biliary cirrhosis ask for an accurate pretreatment diagnosis regarding the degree of inflammation and fibrosis, presence of cirrhosis and its extent. The high miss rate of a blind percutaneous biopsy for the diagnosis of liver cirrhosis has been well-known for years. There is a number of studies comparing the diagnostic accuracy of laparoscopy with blind percutaneous biopsy in chronic liver disease *(table V)*. A metaanalysis of 6 242 patients by Nord *et al.* presented a false-negative result of the blind biopsy from 1% to 61%, leading to a missed diagnosis in one out of 4 patients [6]. These data were confirmed by other groups [5, 9, 23]. In contrast, the false-negative results reported for laparoscopy are in a range of 4% to 18% [6, 23, 24]. Our own results are corresponding to the above-mentioned data with sensitivity rates for diagnostic laparoscopy of 95,2% and histology of 71%, respectively. Similar results were detected in cases with chronic hepatitis-C infection. Laparoscopically liver cirrhosis was evident in 63% of the examined patients, confirmed by histology in 73%.

Table V. Sensitivity rates of diagnostic laparoscopy and histology in the diagnosis of liver cirrhosis

Authors	Year	Laparoscopy %	Histology %
Nord *et al.* [6]	1992	91	75
Pagliaro *et al.* [23]	1983	100	82
Jalan *et al.* [24]	1995	100	94
Poniachik *et al.* [5]	1996	99	68
Helmreich-Becker *et al.* [7]	1998	100	60
Own data	1999	95	71

A prospective study of 100 cases revealed that laparoscopy has a sensitivity of 100% and a specificity of 92% to diagnose cirrhosis [25]. Another study with 434 patients confirmed these results [5]. A false-negative rate for blind biopsy of 32% was demonstrated in contrast to a false-negative rate for laparoscopy of only 0,8% as well. The authors justified this high diagnostic accuracy with the direct visualization of the liver surface obtained by laparoscopy. The macroscopic detection of regenerative nodules, circumferential fibrotic retraction and firmness to indirect palpation seems to be responsible for this high diagnostic yield of laparoscopy [26, 27]. The diagnosis of cirrhosis requires the histological finding of regenerating nodules, perinodular fibrosis and distortion of the hepatic architecture. The percutaneous biopsy frequently offers only small fragmented specimen, leading to the high miss rate of cirrhosis by this method. As a result of these data, the combination of both diagnostic laparoscopy and biopsy under visual control has to be considered as the gold standard in the diagnosis of liver cirrhosis.

Laparoscopy is able to supply the examiner with additional information in patients with chronic liver disease. Not only the direct visualization of the liver surface and the possibility of a guided biopsy seem to be advantageous, also the inspection of both liver lobes and the presence of intraabdominal portosystemic bypasses can be attained by laparoscopy. The aim of one study was to evaluate the correlation of laparoscopic findings and the prognosis of 372 patients with suspected cirrhosis. Tamada *et al.* separated the degree of nodularity from grade I (mild nodularity) to grade III (hemispheric nodules all over surface). They were able to describe a greater clinical value of the laparoscopic evaluation of the cirrhosis in determining the prognosis compared to the histological findings [28]. The size of the right lobe, but not of the left node was of prognostic significance. For an enlarged right lobe a 5 -year survival of 78% compared to 61% with an atrophic right lobe was demonstrated. Additional significant prognostic differences were observed with respect to the degree of regenerating nodules, the formation of small lymphatic vesicles and the degree of splenomegaly found at laparoscopy either.

The characteristics of chronic hepatitis without cirrhosis are more diffuse and homogenous histologic processes. Presumably, the diagnostic accuracy of a percutaneous liver biopsy should be better in these patients than in cirrhotic liver disease [27]. The group reported different histological findings in laparoscopic biopsies taken from right and left lobes in 24% of their patients. In 35% of these a different diagnosis was made, and in over 60% there was a different degree of inflammation between both lobes. Similar findings in both lobes were detected only in 5% of patients. This stresses the need of laparoscopy for this group of patients and shows that a single biopsy from one liver lobe for treatment control is inadequate. Unsuspected hepatocellular carcinoma not detected by other imaging techniques may be detected by additional laparoscopy and lapUS. Kameda *et al.* proposed a significantly increased risk in developing hepatocellur carcinoma associated with the laparoscopic finding of large complex regenerate nodules of liver cirrhosis [29].

Focal liver disease is usually associated with a primary hepatocellular carcinoma or hepatic metastases of other malignancies. The differentiation and evaluation of these patients is another important aspect in the diagnostic spectrum of laparoscopy. As above-mentioned, laparoscopy plays a crucial role in the staging of abdominal malignancies. Laparoscopy is the choice procedure to provide a definitive diagnosis, especially in patients with negative imaging studies and suspected hepatic tumor spread.

Ascites of unknown cause

Laparoscopy proved also very effective and accurate for the diagnosis of ascites of unknown origin. In case of non-diagnosic ascites culture and cytology, additional laparoscopy presented a significant diagnostic benefit in many studies. Peritoneal metastases are usually overseen by other imaging techniques. In our study, peritoneal carcinosis was detectable in 83% of the examined patients. Trujillo *et al.* were able to establish a diagnosis in 89% of their patients, comparable with data from other studies [30, 31]. Due to these reports, the diagnostic laparoscopy has to be considered as the method of choice in the evaluation of ascites of unknown origin and superior compared to explorative laparotomy.

Acute abdomen, abdominal trauma

The diagnostic laparoscopy after abdominal trauma is usually done by surgeons immediately before performing laparotomy in the operating room. The value of laparoscopy to avoid unnecessary laparotomies is broadly accepted today. Recently, there is growing interest by gastroenterologists in diagnostic laparoscopy for the evaluation of patients with an acute abdomen. Many times laparoscopy can be performed directly at the bedside in the intensive care unit under conscious sedation. The introduction of new devices like the "mini"-laparoscopy makes the routine application in this setting desirable. Unnecessary laparotomies of 5% to 40% are reported in patients with blunt or penetrating abdominal trauma. We could assume a substantial decrease of this rate by a wider application of diagnostic laparoscopy.

Conclusions

From the gastroenterologists' point of view, laparoscopy is the revival of an old technique. As mentioned above, this valuable diagnostic tool was abandoned by gastroenterologists twenty years ago because of new and promising imaging techniques which seemed to make the laparoscopy unnecessary while invasive. By now, as we know the shortcomings of the new imaging techniques, we have to learn that laparoscopy continues to play an important role for a great variety of gastrointestinal disorders. Laparoscopy is a valuable tool for the diagnosis of hepatic metastasis, primary hepatocellular carcinoma and peritoneal carcinosis. Furthermore, a more accurate staging of solid abdominal tumors is possible by laparoscopy. Unnecessary laparotomies can be avoided in a number of patients. Laparoscopy remains the gold-standard in the diagnosis of liver cirrhosis. It is superior comparing to imaging procedures and percutaneous liver biopsy. The introduction of new devices will widen its indications. Laparoscopy remains to be an important diagnostic procedure in gastroenterology. It should also be done by gastroenterologists because many of the diseases diagnosed by this technique have to be treated by gastroenterologists.

References

1. Kelling G. Über Ösophagoskopie, Gastroskopie und Kölioskopie. *Münch Med Wochenschr* 1902; 49: 21-4.
2. Kalk H. Indikationsstellung und Gefahrenmoment bei der Laparoskopie. *Dtsch Med Wochenschr* 1935; 62: 1831-33.
3. Classen M, Zillinger C, Frimberger E. Diagnostic laparoscopy: let's do it again. *Gastrointest Endosc* 1999; 50: 297-9.
4. Salky B. Diagnostic laparoscopy: let's do it again. *Gastrointest Endosc* 1999; 50: 299-300.
5. Poniachik J, Bernstein DE, Reddy KR, Jeffers LJ, Coelho-Little ME, Civantos F, Schiff ER. The role of laparoscopy in the diagnosis of cirrhosis. *Gastrointest Endosc* 1996; 43: 568-71.
6. Nord H.J. Biopsy diagnosis of cirrhosis: blind percutaneous versus guided direct vision techniques - a review. *Gastrointest Endosc* 1992; 28: 102-4.
7. Helmreich-Becker I, Meyer zum Büschenfelde KH, Lohse AW. Safety and feasibility of a new minimally invasive diagnostic laparoscopy technique. *Endoscopy* 1998; 30: 756-62.
8. Arnold JC, Neubauer HJ, Zöpf T, Schneider A, Benz C, Adamek HE, Riemann JF. Improved tumor staging by diagnostic laparoscopy. *Z Gastroenterol* 1999; 99: 483-8.
9. Brady PG, Goldschmid S, Chappel G, Slone FL, Boyd WP. A comparison of biopsy techniques in suspected focal liver disease. *Gastrointest Endosc* 1987; 33: 289-92.
10. Brady PG, Peebles M, Goldschmid S. Role of laparoscopy in the evaluation of patients with suspected hepatic or peritoneal malignancy. *Gastrointest Endosc* 1991; 37: 27-30.
11. Warshaw AL, Tepper JE, Shipley WV. Laparoscopy in the staging and planning of therapy of pancreatic cancer. *Am J Surg* 1986; 151: 76-80.
12. Fernandez-del Castillo C, Rattner DW, Warshaw AL. Further experience with laparoscopic and peritoneal cytology in the staging of pancreatic cancer. *Br J Surg* 1995; 82: 1127-9.
13. O'Brien MG, Fitzgerald EF, Lee G. A prospective comparison of laparoscopy and imaging in the staging of esophagogastric cancer before surgery. *Am J Gastroenterol* 1995; 90: 2191-4.
14. Molloy RG, McCourtney JS, Anderson JR. Laparoscopy in the management of patients with cancer of the gastric cardia and esophagus. *Br J Surg* 1995; 82: 352-4.
15. Reed WP, Mustafa IA. Laparoscopy screening of surgical candidates with pancreatic cancer or liver tumors. *Surg Endosc* 1997; 11: 12-4.
16. Conlon KC, Karpeh MS. Laparoscopy and laparoscopic ultrasound in the staging of gastric cancer. *Semin Oncol* 1996; 23: 347-51.
17. Watt I, Stewart I, Anderson D, Bell G, Anderson JR. Laparoscopy, ultrasound and computed tomography in cancer of the esophagus and gastric cardia: A prospective comparison for detecting intra-abdominal metastases. *Br J Surg* 1989; 76: 1036-9.
18. Kriplani AK, Kapur BM. Laparoscopy for pre-operative staging and assessment of operability in gastric carcinoma. *Gastrointest Endosc* 1991; 37: 441-3.
19. Possik RA, Franco EL, Pires DR et al. Sensitivity, specificity and predictive value of laparoscopy for the staging of gastric cancer and for the detection of liver metastases. *Cancer* 1986; 58: 1-6.
20. Bemelman WA, de Wit LT, van Delden OM. Diagnostic laparoscopy combined with laparoscopic ultrsonography in staging of cancer of the pancreas head region. *Br J Surg* 1995; 82: 820-4.
21. Rahusen FD, Cuesta MA, Borgstein PJ, Bleichrodt RP, Barkhof F, Doesburg T, Meijer S. Selection of patients for resection of colorectal metastases to the liver using diagnostic laparoscopy and laparoscopic ultrasonography. *Ann Surg* 1999; 230: 31-7.
22. Schalm SW, Fattovich G, Brouwer JT. Therapy of hepatitis C: patients with cirrhosis. *Hepatology* 1997; 26 (suppl. 1): 128S-32S.
23. Pagliaro L, Rinaldi F, Craxi A, diPiazza S, Filippazzo G, Gatto G, Genova G, Magrin S, Maringhini A, Orsini S, Palazzo U, Spinello M, Vinci M. Percutaneous blind biopsy versus laparoscopy with guided biopsy in diagnosis of cirrhosis. *Dig Dis Sci* 1983; 28: 39-43.

24. Jalan R, Harrison DJ, Dillon JF, Elton RA, Finlayson ND, Hayes PC. Laparoscopy and histology in the diagnosis of chronic liver disease. *Quart J Med* 1995; 88: 559-64.
25. Herrera JL, Brewer TG, Peura DA. Diagnostic laparoscopy: a prospective review of 100 cases. *Am J Gastroenterol* 1989; 84: 1051-4.
26. Helmreich-Becker I, Gödderz W, Mayet WJ, Meyer zum Büschenfelde KH, Lohse AW. Die Mini-laparoskopie in der Diagnostik chronischer Lebererkrankungen. *Endoskopie Heute* 1997; 2: 195-200.
27. Jeffers LJ, Findor A, Thung SN, Reddy KR, Silva M, Schiff ER. Minimizing sampling error with laparoscopic guided liver biopsy of right and left lobes. *Gastrointest Endosc* 1991; 37: A266.
28. Tameda Y, Yoshizawa M, Takase K, Nakano Y. Prognostic value of peritoneoscopic findings in cirrhosis of the liver. *Gastrointest Endosc* 1990; 36: 34-8.
29. Kameda Y, Asakawa H, Shimomura S, Shinji Y. Laparoscopic prediction of hepatocellular carcinoma in cirrhosis patients. *J Gastroenterol Hepatol* 1997; 12: 576-81.
30. Trujillo NP. Peritoneoscopy and guided biopsy in the diagnosis of intraabdominal disease. *Gastroenterology* 1976; 24: 1083-5.
31. Porcel A, Alcain G, Moreno M. Value of laparoscopy in ascites of undetermined origin. *Rev Esp Enferm Dig* 1996; 88: 485-9.

Achevé d'imprimer par Corlet, Imprimeur, S.A.
14110 Condé-sur-Noireau (France)
N° d'Imprimeur : 50202 - Dépôt légal : novembre 2000

Imprimé en U.E.